The Trauma Golden Hour

Adonis Nasr • Flavio Saavedra Tomasich
Iwan Collaço • Phillipe Abreu
Nicholas Namias • Antonio Marttos
Editors

The Trauma Golden Hour

A Practical Guide

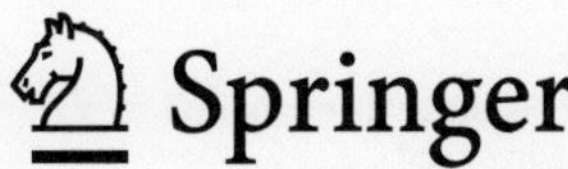

Editors
Adonis Nasr
Federal University of Paraná
Curitiba, Paraná, Brazil

Iwan Collaço
Federal University of Paraná
Curitiba, Paraná, Brazil

Nicholas Namias
Ryder Trauma Center
Jackson Memorial Hospital
University of Miami
Miami, FL
USA

Flavio Saavedra Tomasich
Federal University of Paraná
Curitiba, Paraná, Brazil

Phillipe Abreu
Federal University of Parana
Hospital do Trabalhador
Curitiba, Paraná, Brazil

Antonio Marttos
Ryder Trauma Center
Jackson Memorial Hospital
University of Miami
Miami, FL
USA

ISBN 978-3-030-26442-0   ISBN 978-3-030-26443-7   (eBook)
https://doi.org/10.1007/978-3-030-26443-7

© Springer Nature Switzerland AG 2020, corrected publication 2020
This work is subject to copyright. All rights are reserved by the Publisher, whether the whole or part of the material is concerned, specifically the rights of translation, reprinting, reuse of illustrations, recitation, broadcasting, reproduction on microfilms or in any other physical way, and transmission or information storage and retrieval, electronic adaptation, computer software, or by similar or dissimilar methodology now known or hereafter developed.
The use of general descriptive names, registered names, trademarks, service marks, etc. in this publication does not imply, even in the absence of a specific statement, that such names are exempt from the relevant protective laws and regulations and therefore free for general use.
The publisher, the authors, and the editors are safe to assume that the advice and information in this book are believed to be true and accurate at the date of publication. Neither the publisher nor the authors or the editors give a warranty, expressed or implied, with respect to the material contained herein or for any errors or omissions that may have been made. The publisher remains neutral with regard to jurisdictional claims in published maps and institutional affiliations.

This Springer imprint is published by the registered company Springer Nature Switzerland AG
The registered company address is: Gewerbestrasse 11, 6330 Cham, Switzerland

Foreword

This pocket book entitled *Trauma Golden Hour* is a comprehensive review of trauma care, primarily in the format of algorithms. It is based on the extensive experience of Drs. Adonis Nasr, Flavio Tomasich, Phillipe Abreu, and from the Hospital do Trabalhador/Federal University of Parana in Curitiba, Parana, Brazil, and Drs. Nicholas Namias and Antonio Marttos, Jr., from the Ryder Trauma Center-Jackson Memorial Hospital/University of Miami, Miami, Florida, USA. The Hospital do Trabalhador is now over 70 years old and has had a Trauma Center for the past 20 years. The Trauma Center is one of the busiest in the Western Hemisphere admitting over 10,000 injured patients per year and evaluating another 80,000 patients with lesser injuries or surgical emergencies/urgencies. The Ryder Trauma Center-Jackson Memorial Hospital is now over 25 years old and is one of the busiest in the United States with over 3500 admissions per year and multiple academic contributions to the field.

Trauma Golden Hour is truly a mini-textbook with 5 introductory chapters (history, epidemiology, critical care, injury severity scoring, trauma systems and triage), 35 chapters on clinical management (initial trauma care to management of injuries to organs to violence in children), and concluding chapters on nutritional support and diagnostic imaging. The chapters are comprehensive, but concise, and the algorithms reflect the extensive knowledge of trauma care by the surgeons at the two well-known trauma centers.

This much-needed pocket book will serve as a readily available resource for surgeons in system planning and in the trauma room, operating room, intensive care unit, and beyond. In addition, it will serve as an excellent foundation for the trauma training of surgical fellows and residents, medical students, nurses, and paramedical professionals.

Congratulations to the editors on completing this readily accessible and practical review of trauma care. It will enhance the care of injured patients in the Western Hemisphere and beyond and be another in the continuing contributions to trauma care from the two trauma centers represented by the editors.

Baltimore, MD, USA   David V. Feliciano, MD

Preface

This project originated in discussions between two faculties of surgery from two very different healthcare systems. Two groups from different countries, from institutions with different training principles, resources, and methods, with a common goal: "The premise of high-quality patient care for victims of trauma." This was the necessary foundation to push the present work, a message of support and encouragement to all those health professionals, who regardless of the conditions in the working environment they are choose to dedicate their lives to trauma care.

Both groups understand that the fundamental resource for providing high-quality trauma care is the people providing such care. Qualified professionals with knowledge of the different variables involved in trauma care can overcome all difficulties to provide optimal and compassionate care of trauma patients.

It seems unlikely that two such different institutions would have common aspects to share. This book exemplifies that when the treatment approach is standardized, planned, and humanized, it is possible to overcome the differences in our distinct societies.

Trauma has been present in men's life since the beginning of time and accompanies them throughout the different epochs, shaping the changes of living in society. From the current perspective of the world, it does not seem to us that trauma will abandon mankind, and this encourages both groups of professors to bet on teaching the proper care of this disease in any part of the world.

Despite technological advances, trauma remains a universal critical challenge, regardless of the degree of development and economic power of the society in question. Regions with few resources and others with multiple diagnostic and therapeutic tools face the "Dark Monster" of trauma every day. It uses various characters attacking its victim individually, but causing systemic damage to the entire community.

We conceived of this book so that the readers, independent of the structural conditions of care in which they are inserted, would have a reference of support for the adequate care of trauma patients. There are plenty of textbooks on trauma management of excellent quality. Most of them have a similar format, addressing pathophysiology, diagnosis, and treatment in a sequential manner. Additionally, the use of advaced technology is increasingly referred to as the main tool in the management of trauma. The authors are not opposed to the use of technology, quite the contrary.

But the subliminal message of this project is that: what is most important in the trauma care and the quality of training of the healthcare providers, regardless of the available technical resources.

We were looking for a message different from everything else we had seen. It had to be theoretically correct, with practical application, but in a universal way. Thus, this work introduces readers to the gold standards of trauma care and the feasible alternatives to achieve good outcomes in places with fewer resources, without ever ceasing to look to the future horizon of advances focusing on places with better technology and conditions. This paradox for trauma care, imposed by living in disparate societies, needed an approach with references to both extremes, which will guide the different intermediate shades of care.

Along the journey of editing this book we were delighted to have the chance of working closely together with two outstanding young surgeons, extremely dedicated to the project, especially on the partnership liaison between Brazilian and American contributing authors. Mariana Jucá Moscardi worked on the University of Miami branch of the book, actively participating with the coordination of reviews and improvements with coauthors, while Ana Luisa Bettega endured through a challenging path of translating Brazilian texts into English back-and-forth to overcome the initial language barrier imposed by more than 4000 miles that physically separated the authors from the Federal University of Parana branch.

Thus, the authors intend this work to be a helpful tool for general surgeons, trauma and acute care surgeons, emergency physicians, residents, students, and all health professionals who work in trauma care in different parts of the world, so that the differences between these places are less stressed each day, leading to better results for our patients.

Curitiba, Paraná, Brazil   Adonis Nasr
Curitiba, Paraná, Brazil   Phillipe Abreu
Curitiba, Paraná, Brazil   Flavio Saavedra Tomasich
Curitiba, Paraná, Brazil   Iwan Collaço
Miami, FL, USA   Nicholas Namias
Miami, FL, USA   Antonio Marttos

The original version of this book was revised: The correction to this book can be found at https://doi.org/10.1007/978-3-030-26443-7_43

Contents

Contributors

Marcelo Abagge Department of Surgery, Hospital do Trabalhador Trauma Center, Federal University of Parana, Curitiba, Brazil

Bruna Arcoverde Abbott Iwan Collaço Trauma Research Group, Department of Surgery, Hospital do Trabalhador Trauma Center, Federal University of Parana, Curitiba, Brazil

Phillipe Abreu Iwan Collaço Trauma Research Group, Department of Surgery, Hospital do Trabalhador Trauma Center, Federal University of Parana, Curitiba, Brazil

Department of Surgery, Hospital do Trabalhador Trauma Center, Federal University of Parana, Curitiba, Brazil

Angelo Erzinger Alves Department of Surgery, Hospital do Trabalhador Trauma Center, Federal University of Parana, Curitiba, Brazil

Rodrigo Furtado Andrade Department of Surgery, Hospital do Trabalhador Trauma Center, Federal University of Parana, Curitiba, Brazil

Maymoona Attiyat Ryder Trauma Center – Jackson Health System, Miller School of Medicine, University of Miami, Miami, FL, USA

Camilo A. Avella Molano Universidad de Los Andes, Bogota, Colombia

Renar Brito Barros Department of Surgery, Hospital do Trabalhador Trauma Center, Federal University of Parana, Curitiba, Brazil

Mateus Belotte Department of Surgery, Hospital do Trabalhador Trauma Center, Federal University of Parana, Curitiba, Brazil

Marcel Luiz Benato Department of Surgery, Hospital do Trabalhador Trauma Center, Federal University of Parana, Curitiba, Brazil

Ana Luisa Bettega Iwan Collaço Trauma Research Group, Department of Surgery, Hospital do Trabalhador Trauma Center, Federal University of Parana, Curitiba, Brazil

Alessandra Borges Department of Surgery, Hospital do Trabalhador Trauma Center, Federal University of Parana, Curitiba, Brazil

Luis Fernando Spagnuolo Brunello Iwan Collaço Trauma Research Group, Department of Surgery, Hospital do Trabalhador Trauma Center, Federal University of Parana, Curitiba, Brazil

Thais Bussyguin Department of Pediatrics, Hospital do Trabalhador Trauma Center, Federal University of Parana, Curitiba, Brazil

Caroline Butler Ryder Trauma Center – Jackson Health System, Miller School of Medicine, University of Miami, Miami, FL, USA

Patricia Marie Byers Division of Trauma Surgery & Critical Care, DeWitt Daughtry Family Department of Surgery, Miller School of Medicine, University of Miami, Miami, FL, USA

Patricia Byers Division of Trauma Surgery & Critical Care, DeWitt Daughtry Family Department of Surgery, Miller School of Medicine, University of Miami, Miami, FL, USA

Carlos Hugo Barros Cardoso Department of Surgery, Hospital do Trabalhador Trauma Center, Federal University of Parana, Curitiba, Brazil

Gustavo Rodrigues Alves Castro Department of Surgery, Hospital do Trabalhador Trauma Center, Federal University of Parana, Curitiba, Brazil

Haiana Lopes Cavalheiro Iwan Collaço Trauma Research Group, Department of Surgery, Hospital do Trabalhador Trauma Center, Federal University of Parana, Curitiba, Brazil

Ana Gabriela Clemente Iwan Collaço Trauma Research Group, Department of Surgery, Hospital do Trabalhador Trauma Center, Federal University of Parana, Curitiba, Brazil

Iwan Collaço Department of Surgery, Hospital do Trabalhador Trauma Center, Federal University of Parana, Curitiba, Brazil

Carlos Alberto Bidutte Cortez Department of Surgery, Hospital do Trabalhador Trauma Center, Federal University of Parana, Curitiba, Brazil

Renato da Silva Freitas Division of Plastic Surgery, Department of Surgery, Hospital do Trabalhador Trauma Center, Federal University of Parana, Curitiba, Brazil

Ana Gabriela Clemente da Silva Iwan Collaço Trauma Research Group, Department of Surgery, Hospital do Trabalhador Trauma Center, Federal University of Parana, Curitiba, Brazil

Leonardo Dau Department of Surgery, Hospital do Trabalhador Trauma Center, Federal University of Parana, Curitiba, Brazil

Rafaela de Araújo Molteni Department of Surgery, Hospital do Trabalhador Trauma Center, Federal University of Parana, Curitiba, Brazil

Fábio Henrique de Carvalho Department of Surgery, Hospital do Trabalhador Trauma Center, Federal University of Parana, Curitiba, Brazil

Mariana Vieira Delazeri Department of Surgery, Hospital do Trabalhador Trauma Center, Federal University of Parana, Curitiba, Brazil

João Henrique Felicio de Lima Department of Surgery, Hospital do Trabalhador Trauma Center, Federal University of Parana, Curitiba, Brazil

Pedro Grein del Santoro Department of Surgery, Hospital do Trabalhador Trauma Center, Federal University of Parana, Curitiba, Brazil

Janaina de Oliveira Poy Faculdade de Ciências Médicas de Santos, Santos, São Paulo, Brazil

Marcos Chesi de Oliveira Jr Department of Surgery, Hospital do Trabalhador Trauma Center, Federal University of Parana, Curitiba, Brazil

Jéssica Romanelli Amorim de Souza Iwan Collaço Trauma Research Group, Department of Surgery, Hospital do Trabalhador Trauma Center, Federal University of Parana, Curitiba, Brazil

Maykon Martins de Souza Iwan Collaço Trauma Research Group, Department of Surgery, Hospital do Trabalhador Trauma Center, Federal University of Parana, Curitiba, Brazil

Nelson Fernandes de Souza Jr Department of Surgery, Hospital do Trabalhador Trauma Center, Federal University of Parana, Curitiba, Brazil

Alan Cesar Diorio Department of Surgery, Hospital do Trabalhador Trauma Center, Federal University of Parana, Curitiba, Brazil

Imad Izat El Tawil Department of Surgery, Hospital do Trabalhador Trauma Center, Federal University of Parana, Curitiba, Brazil

Anthony Ferrantella Department of Surgery, University of Miami, Miami, FL, USA

Raphaella Ferreira Iwan Collaço Trauma Research Group, Hospital do Trabalhador Trauma Center, Federal University of Parana, Curitiba, Brazil

José Marcos Lavrador Filho Department of Surgery, Hospital do Trabalhador Trauma Center, Federal University of Parana, Curitiba, Brazil

Márcio Luciano Canevari Filho Iwan Collaço Trauma Research Group, Department of Surgery, Hospital do Trabalhador Trauma Center, Federal University of Parana, Curitiba, Brazil

Enrique Ginzburg Division of Trauma Surgery & Critical Care, DeWitt Daughtry Family Department of Surgery, Miller School of Medicine, University of Miami, Miami, FL, USA

Regina Maria Goolkate Iwan Collaço Trauma Research Group, Department of Surgery, Hospital do Trabalhador Trauma Center, Federal University of Parana, Curitiba, Brazil

Xavier Soler Graells Department of Surgery, Hospital do Trabalhador Trauma Center, Federal University of Parana, Curitiba, Brazil

César Vinícius Grande Department of Surgery, Hospital do Trabalhador Trauma Center, Federal University of Parana, Curitiba, Brazil

April Anne Grant Ryder Trauma Center – Jackson Health System, Miller School of Medicine, University of Miami, Miami, FL, USA

Emanuel Antonio Grasselli Iwan Collaço Trauma Research Group, Department of Surgery, Hospital do Trabalhador Trauma Center, Federal University of Parana, Curitiba, Brazil

Camila Roginski Guetter Iwan Collaço Trauma Research Group, Department of Surgery, Hospital do Trabalhador Trauma Center, Federal University of Parana, Curitiba, Brazil

Rodrigo P. Jacobucci Hospital Universitário Professor Edgard Santos, Federal University of Bahia, Salvador, Brazil

Mariana F. Jucá Moscardi University of Miami, Ryder Trauma Center, Miami, FL, USA

Telemedicine and Trauma Research, University of Miami, Ryder Trauma Center, Miami, FL, USA

Yukihiro Kanda Ryder Trauma Center – Jackson Health System, Miller School of Medicine, University of Miami, Miami, FL, USA

Joyce Kaufman Division of Trauma Surgery & Critical Care, DeWitt Daughtry Family Department of Surgery, Miller School of Medicine, University of Miami, Miami, FL, USA

Zahra Farrukh Khan Department of Surgery, University of Miami, Miller School of Medicine, Jackson Memorial Hospital, Coral Gables, FL, USA

Lúcio Eduardo Kluppel Department of Radiology, Hospital do Trabalhador Trauma Center, Federal University of Parana, Curitiba, Brazil

Edward B. Lineen Division of Trauma Surgery & Critical Care, DeWitt Daughtry Family Department of Surgery, Miller School of Medicine, University of Miami, Miami, FL, USA

Denise Magalhães Machado Iwan Collaço Trauma Research Group, Department of Surgery, Hospital do Trabalhador Trauma Center, Federal University of Parana, Curitiba, Brazil

Andrea Rachel Marcadis Department of Surgery, University of Miami, Miller School of Medicine, Jackson Memorial Hospital, Miami, FL, USA

João Ricardo Martinelli Iwan Collaço Trauma Research Group, Department of Surgery, Hospital do Trabalhador Trauma Center, Federal University of Parana, Curitiba, Brazil

Eduardo Lopes Martins Department of Surgery, Hospital do Trabalhador Trauma Center, Federal University of Parana, Curitiba, Brazil

Antonio Marttos William Lehman Injury Research Center, Division of Trauma & Surgical Critical Care, Dewitt Daughtry Department of Surgery, Leonard M. Miller School of Medicine Miami, University of Miami, Miami, FL, USA

Jonathan Meizoso Ryder Trauma Center – Jackson Health System, Miami, FL, USA

Miller School of Medicine, University of Miami, Miami, FL, USA

Leonardo Lasari Melo Iwan Collaço Trauma Research Group, Department of Surgery, Hospital do Trabalhador Trauma Center, Federal University of Parana, Curitiba, Brazil

Glauco Afonso Morgenstern Department of Surgery, Hospital do Trabalhador Trauma Center, Federal University of Parana, Curitiba, Brazil

Thiago Américo Murakami Iwan Collaço Trauma Research Group, Department of Surgery, Hospital do Trabalhador Trauma Center, Federal University of Parana, Curitiba, Brazil

Acácia Maria Fávaro Nasr Department of Obstetrics and Gynecology, Hospital do Trabalhador Trauma Center, Federal University of Parana, Curitiba, Brazil

Adonis Nasr Iwan Collaço Trauma Research Group, Department of Surgery, Hospital do Trabalhador Trauma Center, Federal University of Parana, Curitiba, Brazil

Jennifer Nguyen Ryder Trauma Center – Jackson Health System, Miami, FL, USA

Miller School of Medicine, University of Miami, Miami, FL, USA

Jean Raitz Novais Iwan Collaço Trauma Research Group, Department of Surgery, Hospital do Trabalhador Trauma Center, Federal University of Parana, Curitiba, Brazil

Carlos F. Oldenburg Neto Department of Pediatrics, Hospital do Trabalhador Trauma Center, Federal University of Parana, Curitiba, Brazil

Marcello Zaia Oliveira Department of Surgery, Hospital do Trabalhador Trauma Center, Federal University of Parana, Curitiba, Brazil

Waleyd Ahmad Omar Department of Surgery, Hospital do Trabalhador Trauma Center, Federal University of Parana, Curitiba, Brazil

Harris Ugochukwu Onugha University of Miami, Miller School of Medicine, Miami, FL, USA

Leonardo Yoshida Osaku Iwan Collaço Trauma Research Group, Department of Surgery, Hospital do Trabalhador Trauma Center, Federal University of Parana, Curitiba, Brazil

Jonathan Parks Ryder Trauma Center – Jackson Health System, Miami, FL, USA

Miller School of Medicine, University of Miami, Miami, FL, USA

Silvania Klug Pimentel Department of Surgery, Hospital do Trabalhador Trauma Center, Federal University of Parana, Curitiba, Brazil

Cristiano Silva Pinto Department of Surgery, Hospital do Trabalhador Trauma Center, Federal University of Parana, Curitiba, Brazil

Louis Pizano Division of Trauma Surgery & Critical Care, DeWitt Daughtry Family Department of Surgery, Miller School of Medicine, University of Miami, Miami, FL, USA

Vinicius Basso Preti Department of Surgery, Hospital do Trabalhador Trauma Center, Federal University of Parana, Curitiba, Brazil

Gerrard Daniel Pust Division of Trauma and Surgical Critical Care, The DeWitt Daughtry Family Department of Surgery, Ryder Trauma Center/Jackson Memorial Hospital, Miller School of Medicine, University of Miami, Miami, FL, USA

Division of Trauma Surgery & Critical Care, DeWitt Daughtry Family Department of Surgery, Miller School of Medicine, University of Miami, Miami, FL, USA

Rishi Rattan Division of Trauma Surgery & Critical Care, DeWitt Daughtry Family Department of Surgery, Miller School of Medicine, University of Miami, Miami, FL, USA

Marianne Reitz Iwan Collaço Trauma Research Group, Department of Surgery, Hospital do Trabalhador Trauma Center, Federal University of Parana, Curitiba, Brazil

Daniela C. Reys University of Miami, Miami, FL, USA

Luiz G. Reys University of Brasilia, Brasilia, Brazil

Thamyle Moda de S. Rezende Iwan Collaço Trauma Research Group, Department of Surgery, Hospital do Trabalhador Trauma Center, Federal University of Parana, Curitiba, Brazil

Márcio André Sartor Department of Surgery, Hospital do Trabalhador Trauma Center, Federal University of Parana, Curitiba, Brazil

Guilherme Vinicius Sawczyn Iwan Collaço Trauma Research Group, Department of Surgery, Hospital do Trabalhador Trauma Center, Federal University of Parana, Curitiba, Brazil

Carl Ivan Schulman Division of Trauma Surgery & Critical Care, DeWitt Daughtry Family Department of Surgery, Miller School of Medicine, University of Miami, Miami, FL, USA

Gustavo Justo Schulz Department of Surgery, Hospital do Trabalhador Trauma Center, Federal University of Parana, Curitiba, Brazil

Seung Hoon Shin Ryder Trauma Center – Jackson Health System, Miami, FL, USA
Miller School of Medicine, University of Miami, Miami, FL, USA

Fernanda Cristina Silva Department of Surgery, Hospital do Trabalhador Trauma Center, Federal University of Parana, Curitiba, Brazil

Alexandre Vianna Soares Department of Surgery, Hospital do Trabalhador Trauma Center, Federal University of Parana, Curitiba, Brazil

Renato Vianna Soares Department of Surgery, Hospital do Trabalhador Trauma Center, Federal University of Parana, Curitiba, Brazil

Wagner Herbert Sobottka Department of Surgery, Hospital do Trabalhador Trauma Center, Federal University of Parana, Curitiba, Brazil

Marcos Takimura Department of Obstetrics and Gynecology, Hospital do Trabalhador Trauma Center, Federal University of Parana, Curitiba, Brazil

Flavio Saavedra Tomasich Iwan Collaço Trauma Research Group, Department of Surgery, Hospital do Trabalhador Trauma Center, Federal University of Parana, Curitiba, Brazil

Gassan Traya Department of Surgery, Hospital do Trabalhador Trauma Center, Federal University of Parana, Curitiba, Brazil

Rached Hajar Traya Department of Surgery, Hospital do Trabalhador Trauma Center, Federal University of Parana, Curitiba, Brazil

Christiano Saliba Uliana Department of Surgery, Hospital do Trabalhador Trauma Center, Federal University of Parana, Curitiba, Brazil

Paola Zarur Varella Department of Surgery, Hospital do Trabalhador Trauma Center, Federal University of Parana, Curitiba, Brazil

João Victor Pruner Vieira Iwan Collaço Trauma Research Group, Department of Surgery, Hospital do Trabalhador Trauma Center, Federal University of Parana, Curitiba, Brazil

Luiz Carlos Von Bahten Department of Surgery, Hospital do Trabalhador Trauma Center, Federal University of Parana, Curitiba, Brazil

Marcelo Tsuyoshi Yamane Iwan Collaço Trauma Research Group, Department of Surgery, Hospital do Trabalhador Trauma Center, Federal University of Parana, Curitiba, Brazil

Beatriz Ortis Yazbek Faculdade de Ciências Médicas de Santos, Santos, São Paulo, Brazil

D. Dante Yeh Division of Trauma Surgery & Critical Care, DeWitt Daughtry Family Department of Surgery, Miller School of Medicine, University of Miami, Miami, FL, USA

Eduardo Zanchet Department of Surgery, Hospital do Trabalhador Trauma Center, Federal University of Parana, Curitiba, Brazil

Nelson Thomé Zardo Iwan Collaço Trauma Research Group, Department of Surgery, Hospital do Trabalhador Trauma Center, Federal University of Parana, Curitiba, Brazil

A Brief History of Trauma

1

Mariana F. Jucá Moscardi, Rodrigo P. Jacobucci, and Patricia Marie Byers

1.1 The Evolution of Trauma

In human life on Earth, the coexistence among humans, animals, and the environment led to a frequent presence of wounds, injuries, and death. In the most primitive times, injuries were frequent, and a mixture of falls and attacks by other humans or animals existed [1].

The history of conflicts and violence between humans causing injuries and deaths precedes around 200 thousand years and persists to this day. The earliest anthropological registry of human violence and the first evidence of intergroup human conflict date back to around 200,000 and 10,000 years, respectively [2, 3]. The admissions in trauma emergency departments nowadays reflect some of the epidemiology of ancient trauma and, despite hundreds of thousand years that have gone by, falls and violence continue to be the major causes of incidents [4].

The added modern reasons for injury are an unequivocal parallel to the development of society, as we comprehend today. Motor vehicle transportation, nonmotorized transportation, and firearms constitute relatively new causes of trauma incidents brought by the development of civilization. Firearms are connected to the discovery of gunpowder, which is thought to have originated in China during the ninth century. However, the use of cannons in warfare was reported only in the mid-fourteenth century [5]. The earliest registries of the first automobile accidents date back to the nineteenth century [6, 7].

M. F. Jucá Moscardi (✉)
University of Miami, Ryder Trauma Center, Miami, FL, USA

R. P. Jacobucci
Hospital Universitário Professor Edgard Santos, Federal University of Bahia, Salvador, Brazil

P. M. Byers
Division of Trauma Surgery & Critical Care, DeWitt Daughtry Family Department of Surgery, Miller School of Medicine, University of Miami, Miami, FL, USA

© Springer Nature Switzerland AG 2020
A. Nasr et al. (eds.), *The Trauma Golden Hour*,
https://doi.org/10.1007/978-3-030-26443-7_1

1.2   The Historical Foundations of Trauma Care

The beginning of trauma care and the beginning of medicine was simultaneous. The primitive physician dealt with injuries in hostile situations practicing primitive preventive medicine, as this was the resource available, where observation, in addition to tentative trial and error, was the most helpful resource. Gradually, a body of knowledge with some evidence-based guidance emerged.

The most ancient trauma care archive dates back to the Egyptian civilization, 6000 B.C., during which time probably the first surgical trauma procedures took place. The Edwin Smith papyrus (1600 B.C.) and the Ebers papyrus (1550 B.C.), which are two of the most important Egypt's medical documents, describe 48 surgical cases containing the treatment of head wounds, topical therapies for burns, and animal bites [8].

The development of trauma care then continues to take place in China and India. In India, the ancient physician Sushruta, 600 B.C., thought to be the father of surgery by many, described over 120 surgical instruments, 300 surgical procedures, and segmented surgery into eight categories [9–11]. Homer's Iliad and Odyssey are the first sources of information about trauma management in the Western world in ancient Greece. Both masterpieces, composed in 700s B.C., describe events that had occurred approximately 600 years earlier. Homer recorded 147 wounds, of which 106 were caused by spears, 17 by swords, 12 by arrows, and another 12 by slings. The Iliad provides what some consider the first written description of the treatment of battle wounds [12–14].

The rise of Greek civilization has been marked as the basis and a turning point in medicine. Hippocrates, 460–377 B.C., considered the father of modern medicine, authored the *Corpus Hippocraticum*, where several injuries, wounds, and treatments were described. Some instances include pus formation that was thought to reduce inflammation of the wound, chest tube insertion for empyema drainage, and tractions of fractures for alignment of bones. The Hippocratic Oath is the earliest expression of medical ethics in the Western world [1, 14].

After Hippocrates, Ptolemy ordered that all world's knowledge should be housed in a library in Alexandria. Greek practitioners took that knowledge to Roman upper classes [15, 16]. The center of medical progress stayed in Rome over the next 4 centuries, accelerated by Galen, 130–200 A.D., who had over 400 writings in which he described suppuration as a valuable part of wound healing.

Humanity continued to engage in battles throughout the Middle Age and Renaissance, and in the last century, with two World Wars, conflicts increased in size and frequency. Conflicts were capable to generate a great volume of injuries that became a fertile ground for the development of care to the injured.

1.3   History and Development of Trauma Care Systems

Because of the intrinsic relationship between trauma and warfare, early trauma systems aimed to provide care for those injured in battles. The Greeks were the first to recognize and provide a system of trauma care. The injured were taken care in barracks or ships, and they used plants as a remedy for the wounds. Following the

Greeks, during the first and second centuries, the Romans developed their trauma system, which consisted of trauma centers called "valetudinaria." There is also evidence of army physicians within the Roman legions.

Another trauma system that aimed to provide care for the military was born in India. In Kautilya's *Arthashastra*, there is evidence that the Indian army had an ambulance service, surgeons, and women to prepare food and beverages and to treat wounds. Indians had a specialized medicine the "*shalyarara*" (surgeon), which meant "arrow-remover." A similar concept emerged from Greece, where the noun "*iatros*," which means physician in Modern Greek, originally meant "extractor of arrows" in Ancient Greek [17, 18].

Military trauma did not have great improvements during the first millennium. It was in mid-second millennium with Ambrose Paré (1510–1590) and Dominique Larrey (1766–1842) that trauma care started to substantially progress for another era. Larrey addressed trauma care in a more pragmatic and logistic way, focusing on rapid removal and treatment of soldiers. To make this possible, he created the concept of "flying ambulance" and brought the hospital closer to the battlefield as a way to operate during the period of "wound shock" [19]. Larrey brought a new concept that is probably a precursor to what later would be known as the "golden hour."

The improvement of trauma care in military combat increased, especially in the nineteenth and twentieth centuries. During the American Civil War (1861–1865), the system of care offered triage, aid stations, and rapid transport to hospitals for injured service members. This strategy set the stage for the management of injuries during the next World Wars and during the Korean War [20].

In 1925, Böhler created in Austria the first civilian trauma system. In the early 1970s, the most notable development of a statewide trauma system occurred in Germany, generating a drastic decrease in road traffic accidents [19]. In 1966, Chicago and San Francisco started the first trauma centers in the United States, followed by the Maryland trauma center, which was the first statewide trauma system in the United States. By 1995, there were five statewide trauma systems in the United States. In 2006, a study by McKenzie EJ et al., evaluating the efficacy on trauma centers based on mortality, showed a reduction in mortality in hospitals that had designated trauma centers [20].

Despite the creation and expansion of trauma centers around the world, prior to 1980, trauma care was at best inconsistent. It was a plane crash in 1976 in rural Nebraska that made it change. An orthopedist and his family were on that plane, and the accident culminated with death of his wife at the scene. The physician and his children had minor-to-severe injuries. The surgeon realized that the treatment offered in the field and in the primary care facility was inadequate. After that tragic experience, a private group of Nebraska surgeons and clinicians identified the necessity of a common language in trauma care, and started a trauma-training program. In 1978, the Advanced Trauma Life Support (ATLS) course was started [21]. In 1980, the American College of Surgeons introduced the ATLS course in the United States and abroad. Nowadays, this program is available in nearly 60 countries and is taught to over one million doctors. ATLS has become the foundation of care for injured patients through teaching a common language and a common approach.

References

1. Matox KL, Moore EE, Feliciano DV. Trauma, 6th edition. New York: McGraw Hill; 2007.
2. Wu XJ, et al. Antemortem trauma and survival in the late middle Pleistocene human cranium from Maba, South China. PNAS. 2011;108(49):19558–62.
3. Lahr M, et al. Inter-group violence among early Holocene hunter-gatherers of West Turkana, Kenya. Nature. 2016;529(7586):394–8.
4. NTDB Annual Report; American College of Surgeons, 2013.
5. Frost RE, Forensic pathology of firearm wounds; 2015.
6. "Le fardier de Cugnot". Archived from the original on 2008-04-16.
7. "Mary Ward 1827–1869" Famous Offaly People. Offaly Historical & Archaeological Society.
8. Rutkow IM. Surgery: an illustrated history. St. Louis: Mosby; 1993.
9. Chattopadhyaya D. Science and society in ancient India (Translated by Gruner B.R.); 1978.
10. Graham H. Surgeons all. New York: Philosophical Library; 1957. p. 35.
11. Lyons AS, Petrucelli RJ. Medicine: an illustrated history. New York: Harry Abrams; 1978.
12. Homer; The Iliad of Homer. (Translated by Richmond Lattimore); 2016.
13. Pikoulis EA, et al. Trauma Management in Ancient Greece: value of surgical principles through the years. World J Surg. 2004;28:425–30.
14. Pruitt BA Jr. Combat casualty care and surgical progress. Ann Surg. 2006;243(6):715–29.
15. Zimmerman LM, Veith I. Great ideas in the history of surgery. Baltimore: Williams and Wilkins; 1961.
16. Davis JH. Our surgical heritage. Clinical surgery. St. Louis: Mosby; 1987.
17. Karger B, et al. Experimental arrow wounds-ballistics and traumatology. J Trauma. 1998;45:495–501.
18. Trunkey DD. The emerging crisis in trauma care. Clin Neurosurg. 2007;54:200–5.
19. Trunkey DD. Trauma. Sci Am. 1983;249:28–35.
20. McKenzie EJ, et al. A national evaluation of the effect of trauma-center care on mortality. N Engl J Med. 2006;4:366.
21. Advanced Trauma Life Support® (ATLS®): the ninth edition. Chicago, IL: American College of Surgeons (ACS), Committee on Trauma (COT); 2012. p. 25–26.

Trauma Epidemiology

Mariana F. Jucá Moscardi, Jonathan Meizoso, and Rishi Rattan

Trauma has long been one of the leading health problems worldwide. Nearly six million people die from injury yearly. Every day, 16,000 people die from injuries, but, for every person dying, several thousand more survive, often with permanent sequelae. Trauma represents around 10% of global mortality and 16% of the global burden of disease [1]. Although men are more likely than women to suffer a fatal injury (men account for two-thirds of trauma deaths worldwide), injury is a leading cause of death for both sexes in all age groups [1].

Trauma kills more people annually than HIV, tuberculosis, and malaria combined, and the overwhelming majority of these deaths, approximately 90%, occur in low- and middle-income countries. The categorization of countries by economic level is made according to the criteria of the World Bank [2] based on 2002 gross national income (GNI) per capita: low income, US$735 or less; lower middle income, US$736–2935; upper middle income, US$2936–9075; and high income, US$9076 or more. If fatality rates from severe injury were the same in low- and middle-income countries as in high-income countries, nearly two million lives could be saved every year [3].

In the United States, trauma is the fourth leading cause of death (accounting for 6% of all deaths) and the leading cause of death among children, adolescents, and young adults aged 1–44 [4]. In the United States, trauma accounts for more premature death than either cancer, heart disease, or HIV infection [5]. Among persons

M. F. Jucá Moscardi (✉)
University of Miami, Ryder Trauma Center, Miami, FL, USA

J. Meizoso
Ryder Trauma Center – Jackson Health System, Miami, FL, USA

Miller School of Medicine, University of Miami, Miami, FL, USA

R. Rattan
Division of Trauma Surgery & Critical Care, DeWitt Daughtry Family Department of Surgery, Miller School of Medicine, University of Miami, Miami, FL, USA

© Springer Nature Switzerland AG 2020
A. Nasr et al. (eds.), *The Trauma Golden Hour*,
https://doi.org/10.1007/978-3-030-26443-7_2

aged 15–44 years, the leading causes of fatal injury are as follows: (1) traffic collisions; (2) interpersonal violence; (3) self-harm; (4) war; (5) drowning; and (6) exposure to fire. Among people aged 45 years and over, the leading cause of fatal injury is self-harm [6]. It is predicted that road traffic accidents will emerge as the fifth leading cause of death in 2030, rising from its position as the ninth leading cause in 2004 [7].

Accurate accounting of the etiology of injury is limited by variations in diagnosis, terminology, and reporting practices for injury by place and over time [8, 9]. Rather, what is known about the overall nature of trauma deaths is based on a limited number of studies conducted in selected geographic regions using coroner's autopsy reports [10–12]. Injuries to the central nervous system are the most common cause of injury death, accounting for 40–50 percent. The second and third leading causes are hemorrhage, accounting for an additional 30–35% and multiple organ failure, accounting for 5–10 percent. The two leading mechanisms of trauma death are motor vehicles and firearms, accounting 29% and 18%, respectively. Nearly one-third (30%) of all injury deaths are intentional (suicides or homicides). Firearms were involved in 67% of all homicides and in 54% of all suicides [5, 13, 14].

It is important to understand that 50% of all deaths occur within minutes of the injury either at the scene or en route to the hospital. These immediate deaths are typically the result of massive hemorrhage or severe neurological injury. An additional 20–30% die primarily of neurologic dysfunction within several hours to 2 days post-injury. The remaining 10–20% die of infection or multiple organ failure many days or weeks after the injury [10, 15]. This distribution demonstrates how trauma systems are ineffective in preventing about one-half of all trauma deaths. Only efforts at preventing the occurrence of injuries or reducing the severity of the injury once it occurs will be effective in reducing the large numbers of immediate deaths [16].

Combined figures from Australia, the Netherlands, New Zealand, Sweden, and the United States indicate that, in these countries at least, for every person killed by injury, around 30 times as many people are hospitalized and 300 times as many people are treated in hospital emergency rooms and then discharged. Many more are treated in other healthcare facilities, such as family doctors' offices and first-aid clinics [17]. However, these figures reveal little about the extent of the injury problem in less wealthy countries. Typically, inhabitants of countries in the developing world experience a greater number and variety of hazards that lead to injury and have fewer resources for injury prevention, treatment, and rehabilitation. In all countries, people with low incomes are especially likely to experience injury and are less likely to survive or recover from disability.

There are notable disparities in mortality rates for injured patients around the world. For example, one study looked at the mortality rates for all seriously injured adults (Injury Severity Score of nine or more) in three cities, in countries at different economic levels. The mortality rate (including both pre-hospital and in-hospital deaths) rose from 35% in a high-income setting to 55% in a middle-income setting, to 63% in a low-income setting [18]. Considering only patients who survive to reach the hospital, a similar study demonstrated a sixfold increase in mortality for patients with injuries of moderate severity (Injury Severity Score of 15–24). Such mortality increased from 6% in a hospital in a high-income country to 36% in a rural area of a low-income country [19].

In addition to an excess mortality, there is a tremendous burden of disability from extremity injuries in many developing countries [19, 20]. By comparison, head and spinal cord injuries contribute to a greater percentage of disability in high-income countries [21]. Much of the disability from extremity injuries in developing countries should be eminently preventable through inexpensive improvements in orthopedic care and rehabilitation. The loss of productivity due to death and disability from injury represents a significant loss of economic opportunity in all countries. The treatment and rehabilitation of injured people represent a large proportion of many national health budgets. Personal loss to the injured and to those close to them is immeasurable.

References

1. World Health Organization. The global burden of disease: 2004 update. 2004; Available from: http://www.who.int/healthinfo/global_burden_disease/2004_report_update/en/.
2. World Bank. 2002.; Available from: www.worldbank.org/data/countryclass/countryclass.html.
3. Department for Management of NCDs, D., Violence and Injury Prevention World Health Organization. Violence, injuries and disability report. 2011; Available from: http://apps.who.int/iris/bitstream/10665/75573/1/9789241504133_eng.pdf?ua=1.
4. Fingerhut LA, Warner M. Injury chartbook. Hyattsville, MD, USA: National Center for Health Statistics; 1997.
5. Center for Diseases Control and Prevention. WISQARS fatal injuries: mortality reports. 2006; Available from: https://webappa.cdc.gov/sasweb/ncipc/mortrate.html.
6. Krug E. Injury: a leading cause of the global burden of disease. 1999; Available from: http://apps.who.int/iris/bitstream/10665/66160/1/WHO_HSC_PVI_99.11.pdf.
7. World Health Organization. Guidelines for essential trauma care. 2004; Available from: http://www.who.int/violence_injury_prevention/publications/services/guidelines_traumacare/en/.
8. Sosin DM, Sacks JJ, Holmgreen P. Head injury--associated deaths from motorcycle crashes. Relationship to helmet-use laws. JAMA. 1990;264(18):2395–9.
9. Israel RA, Rosenberg HM, Curtin LR. Analytical potential for multiple cause-of-death data. Am J Epidemiol. 1986;124(2):161–79.
10. Demetriades D, et al. Trauma deaths in a mature urban trauma system: is "trimodal" distribution a valid concept? J Am Coll Surg. 2005;201(3):343–8.
11. Baker CC, et al. Epidemiology of trauma deaths. Am J Surg. 1980;140(1):144–50.
12. Shackford SR, et al. The epidemiology of traumatic death. A population-based analysis. Arch Surg. 1993;128(5):571–5.
13. Burt CW, Fingerhut LA. Injury visits to hospital emergency departments: United States, 1992-95. Vital Health Stat. 1998;13(131):1–76.
14. Finkelstein EA. The incidence and economic burden of injuries in the United States. New York: Oxford University Press; 2006.
15. Sauaia A, et al. Epidemiology of trauma deaths: a reassessment. J Trauma. 1995;38(2):185–93.
16. Matox KL, Moore EE, Feliciano DV. Trauma, 7th edition. New York: McGraw Hill; 2013.
17. World Health Organization. Injury pyramid. Geneva: WHO; 2010.

18. Mock CN, et al. *Trauma mortality patterns in three nations at different economic levels: implications for global trauma system development*. J Trauma. 1998;44(5):804–12; discussion 812–4.
19. Mock CN, et al. Trauma outcomes in the rural developing world: comparison with an urban level I trauma center. J Trauma. 1993;35(4):518–23.
20. Mock CN, Denno D, Adzotor ES. Paediatric trauma in the rural developing world: low cost measures to improve outcome. Injury. 1993;24(5):291–6.
21. MacKenzie EJ, et al. Functional recovery and medical costs of trauma: an analysis by type and severity of injury. J Trauma. 1988;28(3):281–97.

Critical Care in Trauma

Luiz G. Reys, Jennifer Nguyen, Camilo A. Avella Molano, Rishi Rattan, and Gerrard Daniel Pust

3.1 Introduction

The presence of multiple comorbidities, combined with natural disasters and traumatic accidents, has resulted in a higher complexity of injuries. As a result, there has been an increase in demand for specialized hospital beds and better quality of care for critically ill patients. Intensive care units (ICUs), and more specifically trauma intensive care units (TICUs), have been established to meet the higher level of care required for the management of these patients.

For surgical and trauma patients, intensive care providers need to possess a strong understanding of pathophysiology and the complications that may arise with certain injuries/procedures to minimize morbidity and mortality. The goal of care is to reestablish homeostasis, treat morbidity, prevent complications and mortality, and functionally rehabilitate this subset of patients. To achieve this goal, the

L. G. Reys
University of Brasilia, Brasilia, Brazil

J. Nguyen
Ryder Trauma Center – Jackson Health System, Miami, FL, USA

Miller School of Medicine, University of Miami, Miami, FL, USA

C. A. Avella Molano
Universidad de Los Andes, Bogota, Colombia

R. Rattan
Division of Trauma Surgery & Critical Care, DeWitt Daughtry Family Department of Surgery, Miller School of Medicine, University of Miami, Miami, FL, USA

G. D. Pust (✉)
Division of Trauma and Surgical Critical Care, The DeWitt Daughtry Family Department of Surgery, Ryder Trauma Center/Jackson Memorial Hospital, Miller School of Medicine, University of Miami, Miami, FL, USA
e-mail: gpust@med.miami.edu

© Springer Nature Switzerland AG 2020
A. Nasr et al. (eds.), *The Trauma Golden Hour*,
https://doi.org/10.1007/978-3-030-26443-7_3

intensivist utilizes and coordinates a multidisciplinary, evidence-based approach to ensure that resources are effectively and efficiently allocated to the patients who need them.

3.2   ICU Structures

There are many ways to structure an ICU. Three common structures are a closed unit, an open unit, or a semi-open unit. A closed unit is one in which the critical care team primarily manages the patient. They place all orders and perform all the procedures. Consultants provide care as needed. In an open unit, the primary team continues to manage their patients directly. An intensivist may not be available for consultation. The last structure is a semi-open unit. In this type of unit, both the primary team and critical care team are responsible for patient care. A semi-open unit is staffed by ICU team 24 hours a day, every day. The ICU team manages mechanical ventilation, pain management, sedation, and hemodynamics. The primary team, however, is ultimately responsible for the patient.

Research on ICU structure and patient outcomes often classifies semi-open and closed units as high-intensity physician staffing models. Open units are considered low-intensity staffing units. Data suggest that high-intensity ICU staffing results in decreased mortality of critically ill patients and decreased length of hospitalization.

3.3   Basics of ICU Care

3.3.1   Ventilatory Support

Airway management and breathing are the highest priority when evaluating a trauma patient. Traumatic injuries that result in acute airway obstruction, hypoventilation, severe hypoxemia, a Glasgow Coma Scale of 8 or less, cardiac arrest, or severe hemorrhagic shock may require securing a definitive airway and ventilation. The goal is to protect the airway, improve gas exchange, and relieve respiratory distress.

3.3.2   When to Intubate

A definitive airway is defined as a tube that is placed in the trachea with a cuff inflated below the vocal cords – endotracheal intubation. The decision to intubate is based on three questions:

1. Is the patient unable to protect his or her airway?
2. Is the patient unable to oxygenate or ventilate?
3. Will the expected clinical course lead to a failure to protect the airway, oxygenate, or ventilate?

If the answer to any of the above questions is yes, intubation is usually indicated. However, it is important to note that a patient may still need to be intubated even if the answer to the above questions is not fulfilled.

3.3.3 How to Intubate

The key to a successful intubation is proper planning and preparation to simulate a controlled environment. Necessary equipment includes endotracheal (ET) tubes of different sizes, different airway adjuncts, blades, and laryngoscopes. Airway adjuncts include nasotracheal tubes, oropharyngeal tubes, nasopharyngeal tubes, and laryngeal mask airways. Medications for preinduction, induction, and paralysis should be available. Finally, at least three people should be available to assist with the intubation: one person to perform the intubation, a respiratory therapist, and a third person to either maintain cervical spine alignment or prevent aspiration.

Rapid sequence intubation (RSI) or induction is the gold standard method when intubating. RSI can be broken down into four main steps:

1. Preparation and pre-oxygenation
2. Pre-induction
3. Paralysis with induction
4. Placement

These four steps provide the highest rate of successful intubation and reduce the risk for complications during the procedure.

In preparing for intubation, inspection of the oropharyngeal cavity and airway is important. Foreign objects that may lead to obstruction should be removed. Adequate suctioning is necessary to maintain a patent airway. A jaw thrust and chin lift can reposition the tongue if it is obstructing the airway. Application of pressure on the cricoid cartilage closes off the esophagus to prevent aspiration. Pre-oxygenation with high-flow oxygen is also important during this step. The goal is to delay oxygen desaturation once anesthetics are administered. In addition, the patient's comorbidities should be assessed. Adequate preparation increases the likelihood of a successful intubation.

After the patient is prepared for intubation, sedative and paralytic medications are administered. Preinduction medications are administered to blunt the sympathetic response to intubation. Common preinduction medications include lidocaine, opiates, atropine, and vecuronium or rocuronium, which reduce the fasciculations caused by succinylcholine. A good induction medication is one with rapid onset and offset. Its purpose is to sedate the patient, but depending on drug choice, it may also be an amnestic or anesthetic medication. Common induction medications include etomidate, ketamine, barbiturates, and propofol. Neuromuscular blockade medications, such as succinylcholine or rocuronium, are administered to paralyze the patient. These medications allow for better visualization of the airway and as a result increase the chances for a successful intubation.

After the paralytic agent is administered, the patient is ready for placement of the ET tube. It is important to note that at any time during this process, if oxygen saturation is 90% or less, the patient should be re-oxygenated back to 100%. If the cervical spine has not been cleared, it is important to have someone maintaining cervical spine alignment. If it has been cleared, the head should be extended and the cervical spine flexed to allow for the most linear alignment. The laryngoscope with either a Macintosh (straight) or Miller (curved) blade is held with the left hand. The right hand is used for suctioning, opening the jaw, and placing the ET tube. The blade is inserted into the mouth, sweeping the tongue to the side. It is then used to visualize the glottic opening. Pressure on the thyroid cartilage can help with visualization. The laryngoscope should then be lifted with the force up and parallel to the handle.

Once the glottic opening is visualized, the ET tube is placed and verification is obtained. Placement can be verified with a chest X-ray. The tip of the ET tube should be approximately 2 cm above the carina. Verification can also be made by auscultating lung fields bilaterally or watching chest rise and fall. Most commonly, placement is confirmed using capnography or an end-tidal CO_2 monitor.

In the ICU setting, once placement is confirmed, a mechanical ventilator is attached. There are many different modes for mechanical ventilation. The cycles are based on either volume of gas delivered or the pressure administered to the airway. In a volume cycle, the tidal volume is determined by the ICU team. In a pressure cycle, the airway pressure is determined by the ICU team. The type of cycle and mode used is determined by the goals of care and the patient's condition.

3.3.4   Weaning and Extubation

Complications of mechanical ventilation include pneumonia, lung injury, barotrauma, and much more. As a result, early extubation should be the goal when possible. Prior to extubating the patient, their ventilatory capacity, mentation, hemodynamic stability, oxygenation, and clinical status should be assessed. The rapid shallow breathing index (RSBI) is the average respiratory rate during a 1-minute trial of breathing on room air divided by the average tidal volume. An RSBI of 100 breaths/(min L) or less is predicative of a successful extubation. It is used in conjunction with other factors to determine if a patient is ready for trial weaning.

Weaning is the process of decreasing support from mechanical ventilation until it can be withdrawn altogether. The process is made up of two parts. The first part is where ventilator support is decreased. The second part is where the ventilator is weaned until it can be discontinued and the patient can breathe on his/her own.

There are multiple different protocols for weaning. Our institution prefers to place the patient on pressure support ventilation mode, as this is generally well tolerated. The pressure support is gradually decreased to <5 cm H_2O. Daily, the patient is subjected to a spontaneous breathing trial (SBT), which best determines a patient's readiness for extubation. Once the patient can tolerate an SBT for at least 30 minutes either on room air or on minimal pressure support, the ET tube can be removed on the condition that there are no contraindications to extubation.

3.3.5 Principles and Goals of Sedation

Sedation is a useful tool in the ICU setting and increases patient safety and comfort. Critical illness, anxiety, pain, and delirium can result in significant agitation, which may lead to an increased stress response. The decision to sedate a patient should be made using the Richmond Agitation-Sedation Scale (RASS) (Table 3.1) once the attempts at controlling the causes of agitation have failed.

RASS was created to prevent over- and under-sedation in the critically ill patient. The usual sedation goal score using RASS is 0 to −2 or 0 to −3. Other scales exist, but RASS is the most commonly used one. The decision of which scale to use and the goal score should be made at the institution level to standardize patient care.

Once the decision is made to sedate a patient, interruptions to sedation should occur at least daily to assess the need for continued sedation. This is particularly important in mechanically ventilated patients where over-sedation can delay extubation – increasing the risk of ventilator-associated complications such as pneumonia. Daily interruptions of sedation may decrease the length of ICU days by reducing the number of days on mechanical ventilation.

3.3.6 Prevention of Pneumonia

Trauma patients are at an increased risk of developing pneumonia because of the need for prolonged mechanical ventilation, increased risk of aspiration, lung injury, and/or pain. Positioning, oral hygiene, aiding the clearing of secretions, and pain control can drastically reduce the risk. In addition, for those patients requiring

Table 3.1 Richmond Agitation-Sedation Scale

Score	Agitation or sedation level	Description
+4	Combative	Overtly combative or violent Poses an immediate danger to staff
+3	Very agitated	Pulls on or removes tubes/catheters Aggressive behavior towards staff
+2	Agitated	Frequent non-purposeful movement OR fights the ventilator
+1	Restless	Anxious or apprehensive Movements are not aggressive or vigorous
0	Alert and calm	
−1	Drowsy	Not fully alert Eyes open to voice and maintain contact for >10 seconds
−2	Light sedation	Eyes open to voice and maintain contact for <10 seconds
−3	Moderate sedation	Eyes open or move to voice No eye contact is made
−4	Deep sedation	No response to voice Any movements are due to physical stimulation
−5	Unarousable	No response to voice or physical stimulation

prolonged intubation and mechanical ventilation, the implementation of weaning trials is beneficial.

ICU trauma patients often report that their pain was poorly controlled. Pain in this patient population affects a patient's ability to take deep breaths, mobilize, and clear secretions. As a result, adequate pain control is crucial in preventing pneumonia. Narcotic pain medications are often used. However, nerve blocks and epidurals have been shown to decrease postoperative pain better than narcotic pain medications. In the trauma patient, particularly when rib fractures are involved, this modality should also be considered.

Immobilization of a critically ill trauma patient results in decreased respiratory muscle strength. The inability for deep inspiration due to this weakened state results in the decreased ability to clear secretions and atelectasis. Incentive spirometry facilitates deep breathing using a mechanical breathing device to reduce atelectasis and promote clearance of secretions. To use the device properly, the patient slowly inhales, holds his or her breath for 3–5 seconds, and then slowly exhales. The goal volume is approximately 3.5 L for a healthy male and 2.5 L for a healthy female. Chest physiotherapy utilizes deep breathing techniques, vibration, percussion of the chest, and coughing to expel secretions.

Aspiration of gastric contents and subglottic secretions, as well as poor oral hygiene, has been shown as risk factors for pneumonia, particularly in intubated patients. It is recommended that the head of the bed should be angled at 30°–45° to reduce this risk, as patients placed in the supine position are at increased risk of aspiration. Suctioning of subglottic secretions and the use of chlorohexidine twice daily until 24 hours after extubation to decontaminate the oropharynx are other effective methods at preventing pneumonia.

The above methods are beneficial in both intubated trauma patients and non-intubated patients. However, additional considerations are required to prevent pneumonia in an intubated patient. Studies have shown that the number of days on mechanical ventilation is positively correlated with developing pneumonia. As a result, a patient should only remain on the ventilator for as long as needed. Weaning trials should be attempted daily. Weaning from the ventilator involves decreasing ventilator support to determine if a patient can be discontinued from the vent. Spontaneous breathing trials determine if a patient can be safely and successfully extubated.

3.3.7 Deep Vein Thrombosis Pulmonary Embolism Prophylaxis and Management

A deep vein thrombosis (DVT) is a blood clot in a deep vein, often the legs. Symptoms include unilateral swelling of an extremity, erythema, warmth, and pain. A pulmonary embolism (PE) is a complication of DVT that occurs when a portion of the DVT dislodges and migrates to a pulmonary artery. This can be fatal. Symptoms include shortness of breath, tachycardia, and chest pain.

Multiple factors increase the risk of developing a DVT, including hypoperfusion due to blood loss and inadequate resuscitation, tissue injury, immobilization, and inflammation. It is recommended that chemical DVT prophylaxis be started within 72 hours from the time of injury barring any contraindications. Mechanical prophylaxis, such as sequential pneumatic compression devices and graduated compression stockings, is also used, but it is less effective than chemical prophylaxis.

Empiric doses of low molecular weight heparin (LMWH) and low-dose unfractionated heparin (UFH) are commonly used for chemical DVT prophylaxis. LMWH has many benefits over UFH. First, it can be administered once a day compared to three times daily for UFH. In addition, critically ill trauma patients who receive LMWH have a lower risk of DVTs. For those with reduced renal function or kidney injury, UFH is recommended. Contraindications to chemical prophylaxis include active bleeding and heparin-induced thrombocytopenia.

DVT prophylaxis reduces the risk of developing a DVT, but it does not eliminate the risk altogether. Diagnosis is made clinically and with compressive ultrasound. Diagnosis of PE is made using computed tomography angiography. For patients who are found to have DVT or PE, hemodynamic instability needs to be managed first. Then, therapeutic doses of LMWH or UFH are administered until the patient is on a therapeutic dose of warfarin or a direct thrombin inhibitor, or the patient is started on a direct Xa inhibitor as a monotherapy. For patients with contraindications to chemical anticoagulation, placement of inferior vena cava filters is recommended.

Nutrition: The utilization of fat, protein, and glucose in healing an injury, fighting off an infection, and inflammation results in a hypermetabolic state that puts trauma patients at an increased risk for malnutrition. Decisions on enteral or parenteral nutrition, when to start feeding the patient, and the amount of nutritional support can be difficult. Enteral nutrition is viewed as the more natural route because the patient is fed using the gastrointestinal tract – allowing the intestines to absorb the nutrients. In parenteral nutrition, fat, protein, and carbohydrates are administered intravenously.

In most situations, early enteral nutrition is the preferred route. Patients fed within 72 hours of injury have better outcomes, such as decreased risk of sepsis, pneumonia, intraabdominal abscesses, and multiorgan dysfunction syndrome. Special considerations need to be made for burn patients and those with closed head injuries. For burn patients, enteral nutrition should be started within 12 hours of injury to reduce the risk of gastroparesis. For those with closed head injuries, enteral nutrition should be started once gastrointestinal function has returned, generally at least 3–6 days after injury.

Enteral access can be achieved through a nasogastric tube, a gastrostomy tube, a gastrojejunostomy tube, or a jejunostomy tube. There are multiple different nutritional formulas available for enteral feeding, which will not be discussed in this chapter. Complications associated with this route include aspiration, diarrhea, distention, and bowel necrosis.

Parenteral nutrition should be utilized when there is a total enteral failure or appropriate enteral access is unlikely obtainable within a week from the date of injury. Although parenteral nutrition can be administered peripherally, central administration is the preferred route because the delivered nutrition can be more concentrated and there is a decreased risk of thrombophlebitis. The nutrition administered is a mixture of dextrose, glucose, lipids, electrolytes, vitamins, and minerals. Complications associated with parenteral nutrition include electrolyte abnormalities, hyperglycemia, essential fatty acid deficiency, micronutrient deficiency, deep vein thromboses, and sepsis.

A patient's minimum caloric intake is determined by the basal energy expenditure (BEE), which is calculated using the Harris-Benedict formula.

- BEE for males = 66.5 + (13.8 × weight in kg) + (5 × height in cm) – (6.8 × age in years).
- BEE for females = 655 + (9.6 × weight in kg) + (1.8 × height in cm) – (4.7 × age in years).

Multipliers are then used to account for the patient's stress and activity level. Patients who have been without nutrition for prolonged periods of time are at a risk for refeeding syndrome, which is often characterized by hypophosphatemia, hypomagnesemia, and hypokalemia. As a result, it is important to start a patient at 0.75 × BEE and then slowly increase to the patient's goal caloric intake.

Bibliography

1. Moore EE, Mattox KL, Feliciano DV. Trauma. 8th ed. New York, NY: McGraw-Hill; 2017.
2. Barr J, Fraser GL, Puntillo K, et al. Clinical practice guidelines for the management of pain, agitation, and delirium in adult patients in the intensive care unit. Crit Care Med. 2013;41:263.
3. Silveira PH. Unidades de Terapia Intensiva. Resolução CREMESP n° 71, de 08 de novembro de 1995.
4. Correa LC. Medicina Baseada em Evidências. New York, NY: Mbe; 2010.
5. Norton D, Mason P, Johannigman J. Critical care. US Department of Defense (US DoD). In: Emergency war surgery. Third United States revision. Washington, DC: Department of the Army, Office of the Surgeon General, Borden Institute; 2004.
6. Stephen AH, Adams CA Jr, Cioffi WG. Chapter 21. Surgical critical care. In: Sabiston textbook of surgery. Ed. New York, NY: Elsevier; 2017. p. 547–576.

Injury Severity Scoring

4

Luis Fernando Spagnuolo Brunello, Phillipe Abreu, Gustavo Justo Schulz, Flavio Saavedra Tomasich, Jonathan Meizoso, and Enrique Ginzburg

4.1 Introduction

The injury severity scores can estimate the prognosis and risk of complications after a trauma. They serve as important adjuncts in triage, patient care, and research [1]. Furthermore, they can be used for evaluation of hospital resource utilization and cost-effectiveness studies in trauma [2–4].

They consist of complex mathematical equations in which variable qualitative and quantitative data are standardized and transformed into a single value, which represents the clinical conditions and prognosis of the patient shortly after injury [5].

However, anatomical, physiological, and any other pre-existing medical problems among patients tend to decrease the accuracy of trauma indices, and as a consequence, several indices have been created [6].

L. F. S. Brunello · P. Abreu (✉) · F. Saavedra Tomasich
Iwan Collaço Trauma Research Group, Department of Surgery, Hospital do Trabalhador Trauma Center, Federal University of Parana, Curitiba, Brazil

G. J. Schulz
Department of Surgery, Hospital do Trabalhador Trauma Center, Federal University of Parana, Curitiba, Brazil

J. Meizoso
Ryder Trauma Center - Jackson Health System, Miami, FL, USA

Miller School of Medicine, University of Miami, Miami, FL, USA

E. Ginzburg
Division of Trauma Surgery & Critical Care, DeWitt Daughtry Family Department of Surgery, Miller School of Medicine, University of Miami, Miami, FL, USA

© Springer Nature Switzerland AG 2020
A. Nasr et al. (eds.), *The Trauma Golden Hour*,
https://doi.org/10.1007/978-3-030-26443-7_4

4.2 The Injury Scores

The injury scores can be classified based on three main categories [1]: anatomic, physiologic, and combined.

4.2.1 Anatomic-Based Scores

1. Abbreviated Injury Scale (AIS)

Injuries are classified by tissue damage on a scale from 1 to 6, with 1 being minor, 5 severe, and 6 unsurvivable [7]. The score consists of two numerical components: the "pre-dot" and the "post-dot." The "pre-dot" is a 6-digit scale that corresponds to the region of the injury, while the "post-dot" corresponds to a severity score (1 = minor, 5 = critical, 6 = unsurvivable).

Benefits: continually updated (last update was 2008).

Limitations: Requires specialized training, scores are not objective.

2. Injury Severity Score (ISS)

It provides an overall estimate of the severity of the patient's anatomical lesions. For this score, the body is divided into six regions (head/neck, face, chest, abdomen/pelvis, extremities, and skin/general); each region receives a degree based on AIS, and the three higher grades of the AIS have their score squared and added together to create the ISS score of the patient [3], with a minimum of 3 and a maximum of 75.

Benefits: universally used and easily interpreted.

Limitations: only 1 injury is counted per body region; only top 3 of 6 regions included.

3. New Injury Severity Score (NISS)

This score was proposed to correct an ISS parameter that could underestimate the patient's injuries. Therefore, for the NISS, the sum of the squares of the largest AISs does not consider the body region, but only the three highest AIS values [8].

Benefits: multiples injuries per region.

Limitations: only top 3 of 6 regions included; not widely used.

4. Anatomic Profile Score (APS)

Unlike the ISS, APS encompasses all serious injuries to a region of the body. Severe lesions (AIS $\geq$ 3) are divided into three major categories: head and spinal cord (A); thorax and anterior neck (B); other remaining serious injuries (C).

Benefits: multiples injuries per region.

Limitations: not widely utilized.

5. Organ Injury Scale (OIS)

Developed first in 1987 by the American Association for the Surgery of Trauma (AAST), the OIS is a scoring system which does not predict outcomes, but provides an ordinal scale to organs and body regions injuries and standardizes the descriptive languages of injuries among physicians.

Benefits: standardizes the descriptive languages of injuries among physicians; continuously updated.

Limitations: not useful for patient outcomes prediction; not widely used.

4.2.2 Physiologic-Based Scores

6. Glasgow Coma Scale (GCS)

GCS is used to describe the level of consciousness of a patient. Composed of 3 parameters: eye opening, verbal response, and motor response. Scores range from 3 to 15, based on the best patient response in each category (Table 4.1) [9].

Benefits: wide utilization

Limitations: variation if measured in intubated/sedated patient.

7. Revised Trauma Score (RTS)

RTS comprises a mathematical equation including Glasgow Coma Scale (GCS) score, systolic blood pressure (SBP), and respiratory rate (RR), and has high accuracy in predicting the patient's chance of survival. Ranges from 0 to 7.8408 [10].

RTS = 0.9368 GCS + 0.7326 SBP + 0.2908 RR (Table 4.2):

Benefits: high accuracy in predicting chance of survival.

Limitations: inaccurate in intubated/sedated patients.

4.2.3 Combined Scores

8. Trauma and Injury Severity Score (TRISS)

TRISS determines the Probability of Survival (PS) of a patient and incorporates the ISS, RTS, age (≤55 = 0; >55 = 1), and mechanism of injury (blunt or penetrating

Table 4.1 Glasgow Coma Score

Eye opening	Verbal response	Motor response
1. No eye opening	1. No verbal response	1. No motor response
2. Eye opening to pain	2. Incomprehensible sounds	2. Extension to pain
3. Eye opening to verbal command	3. Inappropriate words	3. Flexion to pain
4. Eyes open spontaneously	4. Confused	4. Withdrawal from pain
	5. Oriented	5. Localizing pain
		6. Obeys commands

Ref: [9]

Table 4.2 Coded values for RTS

GCS	SBP	RR	Value
13–15	>89	10–29	4
9–12	76–89	>29	3
6–8	50–75	6–9	2
4–5	1–49	1–5	1
3	0	0	0

Ref: [10]

Abbreviations: *RTS* Revised Trauma Score, *GCS* Glasgow Coma Scale, *SBP* systolic blood pressure, *RR* respiratory rate

Table 4.3 Coefficients for TRISS score calculation

	Blunt	Penetrating
b0	−0.4499	−2.5355
b1	0.8085	0.9934
b2	−0.0835	−0.0651
b3	−1.7430	−1.1360

Abbreviations: *TRISS* Trauma and Injury Severity Score, *b* coefficients to score calculation

injury), and has become the standard tool for estimating survival probabilities in a trauma patient [11, 12].

$$b = b0 + b1(RTS) + b2(ISS) + b3(AgeIndex)$$

$$PS = 1/\left(1 + e^{-b}\right)$$

where "b" are coefficients which differ for blunt or penetrating trauma, as demonstrated in Table 4.3.

Benefits: good to quality improvements in a trauma hospital, separates penetrating trauma from blunt trauma.

Limitations: cannot be calculated with missing variables.

9. A Severity Characterization of Trauma (ASCOT)

ASCOT was created to address weaknesses in TRISS. It utilizes the Anatomic Profile (AP) instead of ISS.

Benefits: another alternative for TRISS.

Limitations: complex to calculate, not widely used.

10. Trauma and Injury Severity Score Comorbidity (TRISSCOM)

Created to improve TRISS; the TRISSCOM changes the age used in TRISS from 55 to 65 years and also includes eight comorbidities based on International Classification of Diseases (ICD) diagnosis ranges: pulmonary disease, cardiac disease, diabetes, coagulopathy/anticoagulation, neurological disease or dementia, hepatic insufficiency, chronic renal insufficiency on dialysis, active neoplasia of the hematological or lymphatic system, or metastatic cancer [13].

Benefits: reflects the elderly population in trauma.

Limitations: does not take into account the severity of previous diseases [14].

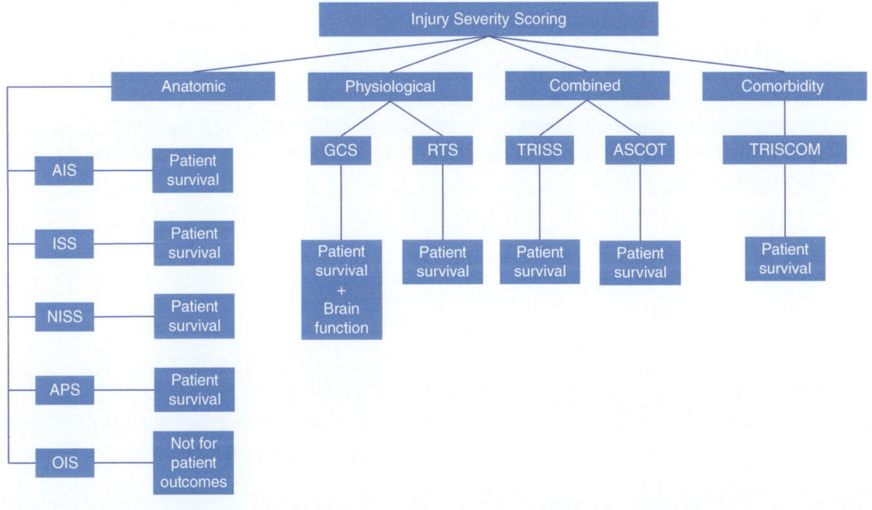

References

1. Mattox K, Moore EE, Feliciano DV. Trauma. 8th ed. McGraw-Hill; 2017.
2. Raum MR, Nijsten MWN, Vogelzang M, Schuring F, Lefering R, Bouillon B, et al. Emergency trauma score: an instrument for early estimation of trauma severity. Crit Care Med. 2009;37(6):1972–7.
3. Baker SP, O'Neill B, Haddon W, Long WB. The injury severity score: a method for describing patients with multiple injuries and evaluating emergency care. J Trauma: Injury Infect Critical Care. 1974;14:187–96.
4. MacKenzie EJ. Injury severity scales: overview and directions for future research. Am J Emerg Med [Internet]. 1984;2(6):537–49. Available from: http://linkinghub.elsevier.com/retrieve/pii/0735675784900810.
5. Júnior GAP, Scarpelini S, Basile-Filho A, de AJI. Trauma severity indices. Med Ribeirão Preto [Internet]. 1999;32(1):237–50. Available from: http://revista.fmrp.usp.br/1999/vol32n3/indices_trauma.pdf.
6. Senkowski CK, McKenney MG. Trauma scoring systems: a review. J Am Coll Surg [Internet]. 1999;189(5):491–503. Available from: http://www.ncbi.nlm.nih.gov/pubmed/10549738.
7. Copes WS, Champion HR, Sacco WJ, Lawnick MM, Gann DS, Gennarelli T, et al. Progress in characterizing anatomic injury. J Trauma. 1990;30(10):1200–7.
8. Osler T, Baker SP, Long W. A modification of the injury severity score that both improves accuracy and simplifies scoring. J Trauma. 1997;43(6):922–6.
9. Teasdale G, Murray G, Parker L, Jennett B. Adding up the Glasgow coma score. In: Proceedings of the 6th European congress of neurosurgery [Internet]. Vienna: Springer Vienna; 1979. p. 13–6. Available from: http://link.springer.com/10.1007/978-3-7091-4088-8_2.

10. Champion HR, Sacco WJ, Copes WS, Gann DS, Gennarelli TA, Flanagan ME. A revision of the trauma score. J Trauma [Internet]. 1989;29(5):623–9. Available from: http://www.ncbi.nlm.nih.gov/pubmed/2657085
11. Boyd CR, Tolson MA, Copes WS. Evaluating trauma care: the TRISS method. Trauma score and the injury severity score. J Trauma. 1987;27:370–8.
12. Champion HR, Copes WS, Sacco WJ, Lawnick MM, Keast SL, Bain LWJ, et al. The major trauma outcome study: establishing national norms for trauma care. J Trauma. 1990;30(11):1356–65.
13. Bergeron E, Rossignol M, Osler T, Clas D, Lavoie A. Improving the TRISS methodology by restructuring age categories and adding comorbidities. J Trauma. 2004;56(4):760–7.
14. The American Association for the Surgery of Trauma. AAST injury scoring scale resource for trauma care professionals [Internet]. Available from: http://www.aast.org/library/traumatools/injuryscoringscales.aspx.

Trauma Systems, Trauma Registries, and Prehospital Triage

5

Luiz G. Reys, Daniela C. Reys, Luis Fernando S. Brunello, Raphaella Ferreira, Phillipe Abreu, and Antonio Marttos

5.1 Trauma Systems

Trauma systems are an integrated, hierarchical, and regionalized network of agencies, institutions, and resources aimed at full collaboration, trained, and dedicated to control, treat, and prevent deaths and permanent disability in a population, directly or indirectly related to TRAUMA disease.

The main objective of trauma systems is to maximize the effort and effectiveness of all human, material, and financial resources available, by covering from prevention and public education, appropriate treatment, and functional and emotional rehabilitation, aiming at full social reintegration of survivors. On the other hand, Trauma Centers (hospital care) provide support and local and regional leadership to trauma-systems, and they can be categorized by levels, which reflect the maturity of a trauma system. They are graded from level I (least mature) to level IV (less mature).

The trauma systems must have multidisciplinary services, coordinated and hierarchical in a defined geographic area, that seek to prevent avoidable death or disability, ensuring inclusive (easy, fast, and efficient) access to patients, in a continuum

L. G. Reys
University of Brasilia, Brasilia, Brazil

D. C. Reys
University of Miami, Miami, FL, USA

L. F. S. Brunello · P. Abreu (✉)
Iwan Collaço Trauma Research Group, Department of Surgery, Hospital do Trabalhador Trauma Center, Federal University of Parana, Curitiba, Brazil

R. Ferreira
Iwan Collaço Trauma Research Group, Hospital do Trabalhador Trauma Center, Federal University of Parana, Curitiba, Brazil

A. Marttos
William Lehman Injury Research Center, Division of Trauma & Surgical Critical Care, Dewitt Daughtry Department of Surgery, Leonard M. Miller School of Medicine Miami, University of Miami, Miami, FL, USA

© Springer Nature Switzerland AG 2020
A. Nasr et al. (eds.), *The Trauma Golden Hour*,
https://doi.org/10.1007/978-3-030-26443-7_5

between all phases. This environment will involve an extensive multi-tasking network with the capability to provide highly specialized and efficient "all patients" conduits and services, especially to those most at risk. Adequate triage in the multiple phases of care for acutely injured patients is needed, prioritizing those at risk of death or disability.

5.2   Trauma Registries

The main objective of trauma registries is to provide information for trauma systems, and that includes accurate and reliable information of the causes, circumstances, and type of injuries of the population. They can be limited to a single trauma-system provider or regional, state, or national providers, and the more integrated they are, the more useful the registry will be for quality improvement of the trauma centers.

The most popular data banks nowadays – with a reliable trauma database registry – are the following five: Victorian State Trauma Registry (VSTR), US National Trauma Data Bank (NTDB), Canadian National Trauma Registry (NTR), UK Trauma Audit & Research Network (TARN), and German Trauma Register Deutsche Gesellschaft für Unfallchirurgie (TR-DGU), with the VSTR and NTDB being the ones most commonly used for research.

In the registration process, information about the cause of death can be obtained inside or outside the hospital, depending on the cause of death. For deaths inside a hospital, the information can be obtained through the death certification. For deaths that occur outside the hospital, a postmortem examination and certification must be performed to obtain detailed information about the causes and the circumstances leading to death.

The advantages of trauma registries are the clinical data collected from the patients; and its importance is well known to hospital database, quality improving, and outcomes research. On the other hand, the disadvantages include the following: (1) The data are collected retrospectively (2). The majority of data collected are in the acute-care admission. 3. They cannot represent the entire population. Besides that, in many low- and middle-income countries, the monitoring of injury-related deaths is not readily available, and that makes it harder to implement injury prevention strategies in those countries.

5.3   Prehospital Triage

Access to trauma victims depends on various aspects. It will be defined by the existence of medical or paramedical services for emergency transport, type of transportation (road, air, or sea-river), hospital resources, and the number of victims. The flow plans and protocols will determine the referral of these patients to the definitive care.

Triage is a dynamic process that seeks to establish, in each phase, a rapid insertion (within 60 minutes) of the patient to a prompt and timely service, adequate to their clinical context and the availability of resources.

It should aim at the best level of care, as well as the definitive treatment, prioritizing the severe patients (estimated in 7–15% of patients), to hospitals of higher complexity (Trauma Centers), often avoiding more medical hospital structures geographically. It also aims to direct patients with less complex problems to hospitals of less complexity so as not to overload the system.

Following are the recommendations (ASCOT, 2006/rev.2011) for field triage and transportation to the highest level of care complexity:

1. Physiological Criteria
   (Glasgow Coma Scale + vital signs: breathing, blood pressure)
   - GSC <14.
   - BP <90 mmHg.
   - RR <10 or > 29 bpm (or < 20 in children less than one year of age).
2. Anatomical criteria.
   - Penetrating lesions of the head, neck, back, and extremities (proximal to the elbows and knees).
   - Open or depressed fractures of the skull.
   - Paralysis or paraplegia of limbs.
   - Chest instability or traumatic deformities.
   - Two or more proximal fractures in long bones.
   - Crushed extremities with grossly impaired tissues, mangled, or without pulses.
   - Traumatic amputation proximal to wrist or ankle.
   - Pelvic fracture.
3. Mechanical criteria related to trauma.
   - Falls.
     - Adults: >20 ft. or 6 m.
     - Children: >10 ft. or 3 m (or 2× ~3× the height of the child).
   - Auto Accidents.
     - Intrusion into the vehicle's internal compartment: >12 in or 30 cm at the occupant's location; or > 18 in or 45 cm anywhere else on the vehicle.
     - Ejection (total or partial) of the occupant of the car.
     - Death of any occupant of the vehicle.
     - Vehicle telemetry data consistent with high risk of occupant injury.
   - Roadblocks: auto vs. pedestrian, cyclist or motorcycle rider or with a significant impact (>20 mph or 32 km/h).

5.4 Special Considerations

- Age.
  - Elderly: risk of injury or death >55 years.
  - Children: should be referred preferably to services that have pediatric surgery or specialized centers.
- When using anticoagulants or with coagulopathies.
- Burns:

- – Without another mechanism of trauma = > triage to Burn Center.
- – With trauma mechanism = > triage to Trauma Center.
- Open fractures; fractures with neurovascular lesions.
- End-stage renal disease requiring dialysis.
- At the discretion of the prehospital care provider (SAMU, EMS).
  Disasters and incidents involving multiple victims.

The only weapon with which the unconscious patient can immediately retaliate upon the incompetent surgeon is hemorrhage. –William S. Halsted (1852–1922).

With terrorism emerging in modern civilian life as an unconventional form of war, as well as an increase in the frequency of significant natural cataclysms (devastating tornadoes, tornadoes, massive floods, and earthquakes in densely populated areas), forced government and medical authorities to provide specific education and adequate training aimed at proficiency in the management of these disasters.

The correct approach requires a coordinated multi-organizational effort in aggressive public policies for crisis management, involving prehospital and rescue institutions, medical doctors, fire departments, police, government agencies, and often, staff military. There should be a dynamic agility in providing easy access to the disaster site, local damage control, crowd control, and adequate information to enable timely and efficient decisions.

In 1970, the US Department of Forestry's Fire Department devised a program of internal control and command structure in crisis situations. Subsequently, many critical concepts were added because of the success of the Israeli Trauma Triage Concept and those conceived and experienced in the later modern military conflicts.

Incidents with multiple victims can be defined as any situation where the volume of patients with injuries exceeds adequate treatment capacity with available medical and hospital resources. In these cases, accurate identification of patient complexity and severity will determine the need for emergency transportation to a trauma center and should be the central mission of any field triage protocol.

In multiple-casualty disasters, prehospital and field staff can use a simplified "simple triage and rapid treatment" (START) approach used for earthquake victims in California:

- Capacity to walking (NO = access respiratory function; YES = nonpriority transport).
- Breath function (>30 bpm = immediate transport; <30 bpm = access peripheral perfusion).
- Systemic perfusion (capillary filling >2 sec = immediate transport, if <2 sec = access level of consciousness).
- Level of consciousness (does not obey commands = immediate transport, obey commands = nonpriority transport).
- Using the "START," patients will be classified into four groups of colors and priorities:

- Red = patients with severe and priority injuries in those who can be saved by intervention, by an immediate and fast transport within 60 minutes; severe impairment of airways, breathing, and circulation; IMMEDIATE TRANSPORTATION.
- Yellow = patients with potentially severe-to-moderate but nonpriority lesions whose transportation may be delayed, as their clinical state is not expected to deteriorate significantly within a few hours.
- Green = minor and nonpriority injuries (a victim with the ability to ambulate and participate in his/her initial care), whose clinical status should not deteriorate over several hours or days; transport late.
- Black = patients dead or with severe lesions and no possibility of survival; palliative care and pain relief.

The great benefit of START is the accurate identification of severe patients who will benefit from efficient and expeditious transportation to the Specialized Trauma Centers, where patients would be assured of resources and better treatment care.

In any scenario, some medical assistance routines should not change in the situations of triage, regardless of the number of patients attended:

- Immediate attention to airways, breathing, hemorrhagic, and circulatory emergencies in a potentially salvageable patient.
- Appropriate handling of pain.
- Systematic evaluation of the patients, although in an abbreviated form, in events of multiple victims.
- Frequent reassessment of patients for changes in clinical status.

Bibliography

1. Moore EE, Mattox KL, Feliciano DV. Trauma. 8th ed. McGraw- Hill, 2017.
2. Briggs SM. Advanced disaster medical response manual for providers. 2nd ed. Woodbury: Cine-Med Publishing, Inc; 2014.
3. Gerhardt RT, Mabry RL, De Lorenzo RA, Butler FK. Fundamentals of combat casualty care. US Department of defense (US DoD). Triage. In: Emergency war surgery, third United States revision. Washington, D.C.: Department of the Army. Borden Institute: Office of the Surgeon General. p. 2004.
4. Lockey DJ. Research questions in pre-hospital trauma care. PLoS Med. 2017;14(7):e1002345.
5. WHO & Monash University. Fatal injury surveillance in mortuaries and hospitals: a manual for practitioners. Geneva, Switzerland: A joint publication of the World Health Organization and Monash University; 2012. p. 7.
6. ICECI Coordination and Maintenance Group. International Classification of External Causes of Injuries (ICECI) version 1.2. A Related Classification in the World Health Organization Family of International Classifications. 2004. p. 1–393.

Initial Trauma Care

6

Mariana F. Jucá Moscardi, Rodrigo P. Jacobucci, Harris Ugochukwu Onugha, and Antonio Marttos

6.1 Introduction

Traumatic injuries can range from minor wounds to multiple organs damage and are the leading cause of mortality globally. Over 45 million people have some kind of disability each year due to trauma [1]. Despite the burden of the disease and clinical relevance, a more systematic approach to initial management of trauma started its foundation only in 1978 [2]. The impact that innovations brought by the ATLS have had on minimizing morbidity and mortality due to injury is undeniable. It still carries a significant public health burden [3]. Worldwide, trauma is responsible for more than three million deaths and 300 million injuries annually, making it a significant, yet preventable global public health issue [4]. With these statistics in mind, it is clear that knowledge of proper assessment and management of trauma patients is imperative in the training of healthcare providers who encounter it on a daily basis.

M. F. Jucá Moscardi (✉)
University of Miami, Ryder Trauma Center, Miami, FL, USA

R. P. Jacobucci
Hospital Universitário Professor Edgard Santos, Federal University of Bahia, Salvador, Brazil

H. U. Onugha
University of Miami, Miller School of Medicine, Miami, FL, USA

A. Marttos
William Lehman Injury Research Center, Division of Trauma & Surgical Critical Care, Dewitt Daughtry Department of Surgery, Leonard M. Miller School of Medicine Miami, University of Miami, Miami, FL, USA

© Springer Nature Switzerland AG 2020
A. Nasr et al. (eds.), *The Trauma Golden Hour*,
https://doi.org/10.1007/978-3-030-26443-7_6

6.2   Preparation

Because of the triad of death of trauma injuries, first described in 1982, which describes the second peak of mortality occurring within minutes to several hours following injury, the assessment and preparation for definitive care are vital. The golden hour of care was the term attributed to the crucial period of care following a complex injury in which rapid assessment and resuscitation are the fundamental principles.

To help prepare the hospital's emergency department, emergency medical services should notify the receiving hospital that a trauma patient is *en route*. Specific information regarding the patient, mechanism of injury, apparent injuries, and vital signs allow hospital-based clinicians to prepare for the upcoming patient care and all the logistics that it may involve.

6.3   Primary Evaluation and Management

In the initial management of trauma patients, ATLS simplifies by using the ABCDE mnemonic (Airway with C-spine protection, Breathing and ventilation, Circulation with hemorrhage control, Disability – neurologic status, and Exposure and environmental control) that addresses five important factors of the patient's condition. First, factors that will rapidly deteriorate and lead to death should be controlled. As an example, airway obstruction and inadequate ventilation are major causes of death immediately after trauma. Consequently, airway assessment remains the critical first step in the treatment of any severely injured patient [2, 5].

6.4   Airway with C-Spine Protection

The very first, and most important, step in the evaluation of trauma patients is assessment of the airway. If the patient is not receiving an adequate amount of oxygen to the lungs, this could lead to hypoxia and inadequate oxygen delivery to tissues. The tissues of the central nervous system (CNS) are of particular concern due to their rapid decompensation in hypoxic conditions.

At the beginning of the airway assessment, it is important to ask the patient their name. This simple question accomplishes two objectives. First, it establishes that the airway is not in any immediate distress. Second, if the patient replies with a logical response, it shows that their current mental condition is relatively stable. Establishing the presence of an upper airway obstruction in an acute trauma is a top priority. The tongue, blood, foreign bodies, and teeth are some of the most common causes of obstruction, which can be identified through signs such as stridor, gurgling, and hoarseness. The patient should also be closely examined for external trauma such as facial, mandibular, or neck trauma that has potential to compromise the airway and lead to obstruction.

The ultimate goal of the airway assessment is to determine if it is necessary to establish a definitive airway (placement of an endotracheal tube). Once it is determined that the airway is sufficiently compromised, immediate action must be taken to maintain the airway. Indications for this procedure include airway obstruction, severe shock, combativeness requiring sedation for comprehensive evaluation, risk for aspiration, severe maxillofacial fractures, and Glasgow Coma Scale (GCS) 8 or lower. It is generally best to intubate prematurely when in doubt, principally in patients with hemodynamic instability, or those with injuries to face and neck that might make intubation difficult due to altered anatomy.

If orotracheal intubation is not possible, then it might be necessary to create a surgical airway through a cricothyroidectomy.

6.5 Breathing and Ventilation

Once airway patency is ensured, it is safe to proceed to assessment of oxygenation and ventilation. The initial assessment process in the evaluation of breathing and ventilation includes inspection, palpation, and auscultation. It is important that this evaluation is done over the neck, thoracic region, upper abdomen, and back. There are many issues that could become apparent during this portion of the exam: simple pneumothorax, penetrating injuries, massive hemothorax, flail chest, etc. However, tension pneumothorax is one of the more emergent abnormalities that may be elucidated. Patients exhibiting signs of tension pneumothorax should be treated presumptively with decompression before obtaining imaging. Delays to obtain a portable chest radiograph can cause significant morbidity. If confirmation is needed prior to treatment, ultrasound can be performed rapidly at the bedside, and it is more sensitive than plain radiograph for detecting pneumothorax [7].

Tube thoracostomy in an unstable trauma patient is positioned in anticipation of both hemothorax and pneumothorax using a chest tube of at least 32 French in diameter. It is placed in the mid- or anterior-axillary line, usually in the fourth or fifth intercostal space.

Although it is meant to monitor ventilation, a pulse oximeter should be applied to the patient as early as possible in order to monitor for hypoxemia. However, there are limitations to what can be discerned from the pulse oximeter. Peripheral vasoconstriction, carbon monoxide poisoning, and rapidly changing oxygen levels are all reasons why the pulse oximetry readings may be inaccurate [6].

6.6 Circulation with Hemorrhage Control

Many patients presenting in a trauma situation will likely have some type of blood loss. Unless it is properly controlled, a hemorrhaging patient can quickly progress to hypovolemic shock, which is why hemorrhage is the leading cause of preventable death after injury. The clinical signs of shock can range from tachycardia and dyspnea to mental status changes and decreased pulse pressure. ATLS [2] recommends monitoring the patient's overall blood loss using vital signs. Therefore, the most important step here is to determine the source of bleeding and control it.

If severe bleeding is noted upon patient presentation, two large bore intravenous lines are placed and pressure is applied directly to the bleeding sight. While this is being done, the patient must also be assessed for bleeding that is not readily noticeable: penetrating cardiac injury, abdominal and pelvic bleeding, long bone fractures, etc. Chest radiographs, pelvic plain film radiograph, and focused abdominal sonographic examination for trauma (FAST) can all be very useful in identifying sources of internal bleeding.

In situations of severe blood loss, it is also very important to consider the need for rapid volume replacement, which can be started once IV access is established. The need for packed red blood cells (PRBC), fresh frozen plasma (FFP), and platelets is determined based on the severity of shock and should be started as earlier as possible in grade III or IV shock. It is important to avoid too much saline before considering blood products. Usually, 1 or 2 L of saline is more than enough. Keeping an eye on the patient's vitals, urine output, and mental status will allow the clinicians to know if they have given the right amount of fluid replacement. In the absence of type-specific blood, O-positive blood is given to men and O-negative blood is given to women.

6.7 Disability: Neurological Status

In the disability portion of the initial assessment, the patient's level of consciousness, pupillary size and reaction, and spinal cord injury level are all evaluated. The main tool for this assessment is the Glasgow Coma Scale (GCS), which tests three areas of neurologic function: eye opening, verbal response, and best motor response. The eyes are a particularly significant point of focus in this exam because it is possible to detect a lateralizing brain lesion by observing abnormal pupillary size, asymmetry, or reaction to light. This neurologic exam is meant to be brief due to the fact that a "complete and detailed neurologic examination is not accurate or warranted until the patient is hemodynamically stable."

6.8 Exposure and Environmental Control

In order to thoroughly assess the condition of a trauma patient, it is very important that they are completely exposed. This means that their clothing must be completely removed. While this allows for a more complete and adequate evaluation, one must also recognize that prolonged exposure places the patient at risk for hypothermia. Many steps can be taken to prevent the onset of hypothermia: warmed air, fluids, oxygen, and blankets. It is also beneficial to infuse all IV fluids through a fluid warmer in order to avoid hypothermia induced by cold fluid administration. The temperature of the patient should be reassessed frequently during the initial assessment.

References

1. World Health Organization. Global burden of disease. www.who.int/healthinfo/global_burden_disease/en/.
2. American College of Surgeons Committee on Trauma. Advanced Trauma life support (ATLS) student course manual. 9th ed. Chicago: American College of Surgeons; 2012.
3. Sidwell R, Matar MM, Sakran JV. Trauma education and prevention. Surg Clin North Am. 2017;97(5):1185–97.
4. Ray JM, Cestero RF. Initial management of the trauma patient. Atlas Oral Maxillofac Surg Clin North Am. 2013;21(1):1–7.
5. Newgard CD, et al. Emergency medical services intervals and survival in trauma: assessment of the "golden hour" in a north American prospective cohort. Ann Emerg Med. 2010;55(3):235. Epub 2009 Sep 23
6. Moore EE, Feliciano DV, Mattox KL. Trauma. New York: McGraw-Hill Education; 2017.
7. Raja AS, Jacobus CH. How accurate is ultrasonography for excluding pneumothorax? Ann Emerg Med. 2013;61(2):207. Epub 2012 Jul 27

Airway Management

João Victor Pruner Vieira, Angelo Erzinger Alves, Fernanda Cristina Silva, Mariana F. Jucá Moscardi, and Antonio Marttos

According to thanatology, the scientific study of death, the emergency patient care is particular since it demands attention to factors that can lead the patient to death, even before considering the causes that brought him/her to the emergency service. In trauma victims, inadequate supply of oxygen to the brain and other structure is the fastest factor that can lead to death, regardless of the etiology; therefore, the assessment of airway stability and ventilation capacity should receive top priority in the initial care of these patients. In all cases, cervical spine must be kept stable as well as assisted ventilation with a mask provided with a one-way valve and oxygen reservoir must be offered.

Patients who arrive in the emergency service in apnea or with reduced level of consciousness should be approached immediately with airway management maneuvers such as head-tilt chin lift and jaw-thrust, procedures performed to prevent hypopharynx obstruction by the patient's tongue. Many times, these simple maneuvers ensure airway patency and relieve hypoxemia. However, on many occasions, the airway must be guaranteed by endotracheal intubation or by performing a surgical airway.

J. V. P. Vieira
Iwan Collaço Trauma Research Group, Department of Surgery, Hospital do Trabalhador Trauma Center, Federal University of Parana, Curitiba, Brazil

A. E. Alves · F. C. Silva
Department of Surgery, Hospital do Trabalhador Trauma Center, Federal University of Parana, Curitiba, Brazil

M. F. Jucá Moscardi (✉)
University of Miami, Ryder Trauma Center, Miami, FL, USA

A. Marttos
William Lehman Injury Research Center, Division of Trauma & Surgical Critical Care, Dewitt Daughtry Department of Surgery, Leonard M. Miller School of Medicine Miami, University of Miami, Miami, FL, USA

© Springer Nature Switzerland AG 2020
A. Nasr et al. (eds.), *The Trauma Golden Hour*,
https://doi.org/10.1007/978-3-030-26443-7_7

In these cases, in which an intervention is required, particular attention should always be paid for basic care in performing the procedure, such as positioning the endotracheal tube adequately with an inflated balloon. The tube should also be linked to an assisted ventilation system with supplementary oxygen.

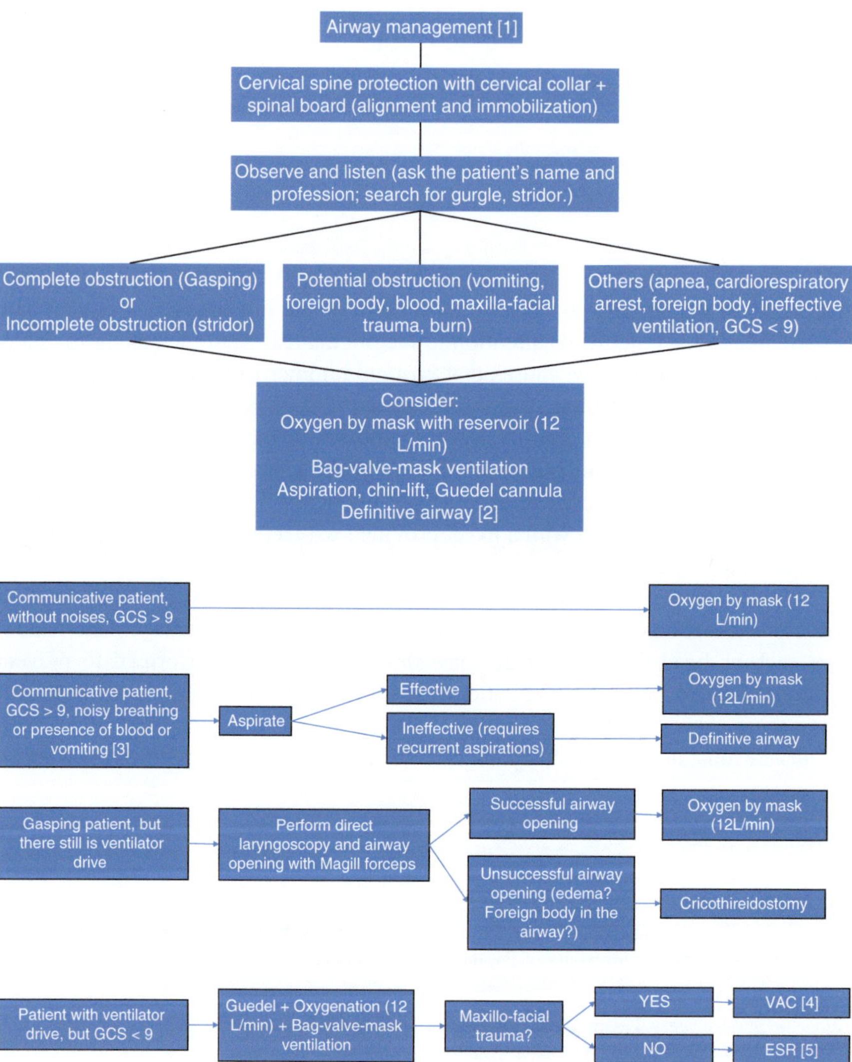

7.1   Conclusion

(1) It can be helpful to perform the LEMON method proposed by the eighth ATLS
    edition, which predicts a difficult orotracheal intubation and is based on (a)
    external inspection; (b) anatomical relations of the axis pharynx-larynx-mouth;
    (c) Mallampati's classification; (e) neck mobility.
(2) The first option is cricothyroidotomy. However, patients with laryngeal trauma
    could require a tracheostomy, which will stabilize the airway below the lesion
    level.
(3) Suggestive of potential airway obstruction or partial obstruction.
(4) Surgical airway.
(5) Rapid sequence intubation (RSI) is a fast and effective method of performing
    endotracheal intubation with prior sedation of the patient, which is based on
    five steps: (a) preparation of the patient, intubation equipment, and materials
    required to perform an emergency surgical airway if needed; (b) pre-oxygenation
    of the patient; (c) medication of the patient with intravenous sedatives such as
    midazolam (0.1–0.5 mg/kg) or even opioids such as fentanyl (2–3 mcg/kg); (d)
    paralysis of the patient with intravenous neuromuscular blockers such as suc-
    cinylcholine (0.5–0.6 mg/kg) or rocuronium (0.06 mg/kg); (e) positioning of
    the tube.

Bibliography

1. Vias aéreas e Ventilação. Advanced Trauma Life Support® (ATLS®)- Suporte avançado de
   vida no trauma. 8ᵉed. 2008. Chicago, IL: American College of Surgeons (ACS), Committee on
   Trauma (COT). p. 43–53.
2. Mills TJ, Deblieux P. Emergency airway management in the adult with direct airway trauma.
   In: Walls RM, editor. UpToDate. Waltham: UpToDate, Inc; 2012.
3. Brown CA. The decision to intubate. In: Walls RM, editor. UpToDate. Waltham: UpToDate,
   Inc; 2012.
4. Bair AE. Rapid Sequence Intubation in adults. In: Walls RM, editor. UpToDate. Waltham:
   UpToDate, Inc; 2012.

Management of Shock

8

Ana Luísa Bettega, Phillipe Abreu,
Wagner Herbert Sobottka, Adonis Nasr,
and Antonio Marttos

8.1 Introduction

Shock is a syndrome caused by a disorder in systemic perfusion leading to cellular hypoxia, inadequate tissue oxygenation, and organic dysfunction.

To approach the shock, the following sequence must be followed: recognize its presence, preferably in the initial phase; establish measures of general support; establish the etiology of the shock; and establish early correction of the primary cause (*stop the bleeding*).

During the establishment of a state of shock, there is a decrease in vagal tone, by stimulation of the baroreceptors, and increase in the activity of the sympathetic nervous system with release of catecholamines; this provides an increase in heart rate (positive cardiac inotropic activity), leading to tachycardia reflex (earlier response), and cutaneous vasoconstriction. In addition, there is an inadequate perfusion of the central nervous system and kidneys, sparing vital organs. This is the initial compensatory mechanism. Therefore, during a care in the emergency room, to evaluate these signs quickly and efficiently, one should observe the *pulse, skin*

A. L. Bettega · P. Abreu (✉) · A. Nasr
Iwan Collaço Trauma Research Group, Department of Surgery, Hospital do Trabalhador Trauma Center, Federal University of Parana, Curitiba, Brazil

W. H. Sobottka
Department of Surgery, Hospital do Trabalhador Trauma Center,
Federal University of Parana, Curitiba, Brazil

A. Marttos
William Lehman Injury Research Center, Division of Trauma & Surgical Critical Care,
Dewitt Daughtry Department of Surgery, Leonard M. Miller School of Medicine Miami,
University of Miami, Miami, FL, USA

© Springer Nature Switzerland AG 2020
A. Nasr et al. (eds.), *The Trauma Golden Hour*,
https://doi.org/10.1007/978-3-030-26443-7_8

color, and *level of consciousness.* Other signs of shock are oliguria (diuresis <20 ml/h), hypotension (systolic BP <90 mmHg or 30% below baseline BP), tachypnea, hypothermia, and reduction of pulse pressure (difference between systolic and diastolic BP).

There are several types of shock: hemorrhagic, neurogenic, cardiogenic, septic, and obstructive (hypertensive pneumothorax).

8.2 Hemorrhagic Shock

It is the most common type of shock in the traumatized patient. It occurs when the presence of bleeding exceeds normal compensatory mechanisms, compromising oxygenation and tissue perfusion. Situations that have significant potential to cause hemorrhagic shock are intraperitoneal, retroperitoneal, thoracic, long bone, and pelvic fractures. If the patient shows signs of shock, it should be treated as hemorrhagic, since besides being the most common etiology, the other types of shock initially respond to volume replacement. *The diagnosis and treatment must occur almost simultaneously.* The initial interventions are based on hemorrhage control, obtaining two calibrated venous accesses and fluid replacement. The patient's response will be used as a guide for volume replacement and for subsequent therapy (Table 8.1). Another measure that may help in the recognition of shock, guidance of volume replacement, and therapeutic decisions is the classification of functional class bleeding (Table 8.2).

Table 8.1 Responses to initial fluid resuscitation[a]

	Rapid response	Transient response	Minimal or no response
Vital signs	Return to normal	Transient improvement, recurrence of decreased blood pressure and increased heart rate	Remain abnormal
Estimated blood loss	Minimal (<15%)	Moderate and ongoing (15%–40%)	Severe (>40%)
Need for blood	Low	Moderate to high	Immediate
Blood preparation	Type and crossmatch	Type-specific	Emergency blood release
Need for operative intervention	Possibly	Likely	Highly likely
Early presence of surgeon	Yes	Yes	Yes

[a]Isotonic crystalloid solution, up to 1000 mL in adults and 20 mL/kg in children

Table 8.2 Physiologic response of hemorrhage by class

	Class I	Class II	Class III	Class IV
Approximate blood loss	<15%	15–30%	31–40%	>40%
Heart rate	Normal	Normal/↑	↑	↑/↑↑
Blood pressure	Normal	Normal	Normal/↓	↓
Respiratory rate	Normal	Normal	Normal/↑	↑
Urine output	Normal	Normal	↓	↓↓
Glasgow Coma Scale	Normal	Normal	↓	↓
Base deficit	0 to −2	−2 to −6	−6 to −10	−10 or less
Need for blood transfusion	Monitor	Possible	Yes	Massive transfusion protocol

Ref.: ACS-COT, ATLS 10th ed

8.3 Neurogenic Shock

It occurs when there is a spinal cord injury and this leads to a state of hypotension due to loss of sympathetic tone. It presents with arterial hypotension without cutaneous vasoconstriction (the skin does not become cold) and tachycardia. The initial treatment consists of volumetric replacement. Remember that isolated head injury does not cause shock.

8.4 Septic Shock

It is a type of distributive shock, in which there is damage to the distribution and blood flow. It is not uncommon to occur soon after the trauma. It should be suspected in situations that the patient takes to reach the hospital and in abdominal penetrating lesions with peritoneal contamination by intestinal contents. The clinical picture is similar to the hemorrhagic shock and should be treated initially with volume replacement.

8.5 Cardiogenic Shock

It occurs in situations where myocardial dysfunction is present. It has several causes such as AMI, arrhythmias, cardiac structural lesions, cardiac tamponade, blunt heart trauma, and hypertensive pneumothorax. Patients with blunt trauma in the chest need cardiac monitoring and CPK dosing. Cardiac tamponade should be always suspected when there is presence of engorged jugular, muffled heart sounds, tachycardia, and hypotension refractory to volume replacement. It is also initially conducted with fluid replacement.

8.6 Obstructive Shock (Hypertensive Pneumothorax)

It occurs when there is unidirectional air leakage into the pleural space, due to injury to the chest wall and/or pulmonary parenchyma. Pulmonary atelectasis occurs with deviation of mediastinal structures to the opposite side, compressing the cardiac chambers and hindering venous return. It is recognized by the presence of engorged jugular, tracheal deviation, subcutaneous emphysema, acute respiratory insufficiency, absence of vesicular murmur, and tympanism to percussion. It is a surgical emergency and should be treated with insertion of a calibrated needle in the 2nd intercostal space in the hemiclavicular line for immediate decompression and posterior closed chest drainage.

8.7 Algorithm

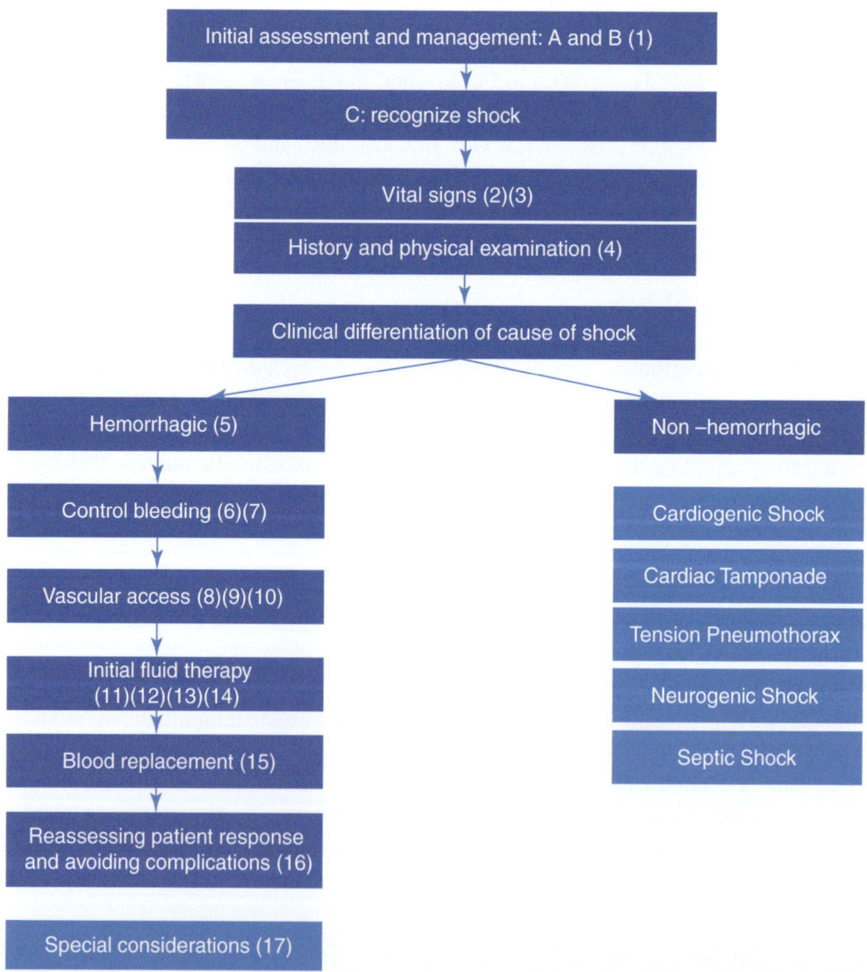

8.8   Conclusion

(1) When in E (exposure): prevent hypothermia which worsens the blood loss by contributing to coagulopathy and acidosis.

(2) HR, pulse character, RR, skin perfusion, pulse pressure. Remember that the normal HR varies according to age.

(3) Obtain hemoglobin and hematocrit, other than serial measurements of lactate and base deficit.

(4) X-ray and FAST can confirm the cause of shock, but should not delay appropriate resuscitation.

(5) Most common cause of shock in trauma patients.

(6) Evaluate external wounds and possible hidden sources of bleeding. Remember that fractures and major soft-tissue injuries can compromise the hemodynamic status of injured patients.

(7) Estimate the amount of blood loss (blood loss can be underestimated from soft-tissue injury, particularly in obese and elderly individuals) (Table 8.2∗), because these clinical signs serve to guide initial therapy. Subsequent volume replacement is determined by the patient's response to therapy (Table 8.1).

(8) Is best accomplished by inserting two large-caliber (minimum of 18-gauge in an adult) peripheral intravenous catheters. The most desirable sites are the forearms and the antecubital vein. The second option is intraosseous and the third is central venous access.

(9) Blood samples for type and crossmatch, appropriate laboratory analyses, toxicology studies, pregnancy testing, and blood gas analysis.

(10) Evaluate tissue perfusion. Gastric decompression in unconscious patients by inserting a nasal or oral tube can avoid hypotension or cardiac dysrhythmia, usually bradycardia from excessive vagal stimulation. Bladder catheterization allows clinicians to assess the urine for hematuria, monitoring urine output, and evaluation of renal perfusion.

(11) Administer an initial warmed fluid bolus of isotonic fluid (1 L in adults or 20/mL/kg in children) – Remember that this includes previous pre-hospitalar administration of fluids.

(12) If shock does not respond to initial crystalloid fluid bolus, look for a source of ongoing blood loss: "floor" and four more (abdomen/pelvis, retroperitoneum, thorax, and extremities).

(13) Absolute volume resuscitation should be based on patient's response to fluid administration. The parameters include urinary output, base deficit, and lactate. The patterns of response are as follows: rapid, transient, and minimal/no response. For the last two, blood replacement is required.

(14) Permissive hypotension.

(15) Is used to transient and to minimal/no response patterns of response to fluid replacement. Consider the type of blood, prevent hypothermia, autotransfusion, massive transfusion, coagulopathy, and calcium administration.

(16) Continued hemorrhage, monitoring, and recognition of other problems.

(17) Advanced age, pregnancy, medications, hypothermia, athletes, presence of pacemaker, or implantable cardioverter-defibrillator.

* Regarding the classification system, consider confounding factors, such as age, severity of injury, particularly the type and anatomic location of injury, time lapse between injury and initiation of treatment, prehospital fluid therapy, and medications used for chronic conditions.

Bibliography

1. American College of Surgeons. ACS. Committee on Trauma Advanced Trauma Life Support. Instructor manual. 10th ed. Chicago: American College of Surgeons; 2018.
2. Townsend C. Tratado de Cirurgia v. 1. 18ª Ed Seção I, Cap 5: Choque, eletrólitos e fluidos. São Paulo: Elsevier; 2007.
3. Curry N, Hopewell S, Dorée C, Hyde C, Brohi K, Stanworth S. The acute management of trauma hemorrhage: a systematic review of randomized controlled trial. Crit Care. 2011;15(2):R92.
4. Parreira JG, Soldá SC, Rasslan S. Análise dos Indicadore de Hemorragia Letal em Vítimas de Trauma Penetrante de Tronco admitidas em choque: um método objetivo para selecionar os candidatos ao "controle de danos". Rev Col Bras Cir. 2002;29(5)
5. Rocha RM. Abordagem Inicial do Choque. Rev Socer J. 2001;XIV(2 Abr/Mai/).
6. Kaur P, Basu S, Kaur G, Kaur R. Transfusion protocol in trauma. J Emerg Trauma Shock. 2011;4(1):103–8.
7. Marson F, Junior GAP, Filho AP, Filho AB. A síndrome do choque circulatório, vol. 31. Ribeirão Preto: Medicina. p. 369–79, jul./set. 1998. Simpósio: Medicina Intensiva: I. Infecção e Choque.
8. D'Ávila AR. Manejo do Choque Hipovolêmico no Paciente Traumatizado. Mom. & Perspec. Saúde – Porto Alegre – V. 14 - n° 1/2 – jan/dez – 2001.
9. Júnior GAP, Lovato WJ, Carvalho JB, Horta MFV. Abordagem Geral Trauma Abdominal. Medicina, Ribeirão Preto. 2007;40(4):518–30, out./dez. Simpósio: Cirurgia de Urgência e Trauma – 2ª Parte.
10. Feliciano DV, Burch JM, Spjut-Patrianely V, Mattox KL, Jordan GL Jr. Abdominal gunshot wounds. An urban trauma center's experience with 300 consecutive patients. Ann Surg. 1988;208:362–70.

Resuscitative Thoracotomy in Emergency Department

9

Mariana F. Jucá Moscardi, Luis Fernando Spagnuolo Brunello, Flavio Saavedra Tomasich, and Gerrard Daniel Pust

9.1 Introduction

The emergency department thoracotomy (EDT) is still one of the most controversial procedures being performed in the emergency department by physicians and the decision to – or not to – do it, is based on the last chance of survival of the trauma victim [1]. The survival predictors depend on the trauma mechanism, anatomic injury location, and degree of physiologic derangement after performing a closed-chest cardiopulmonary resuscitation (CPR). The main objectives of EDT are to avoid the cardiovascular collapse from mechanical sources or extreme hypovolemia, in patients in extremis [1, 2].

The indication after penetrating thoracic injury is to perform in every pulseless patient or profound refractory shock. In case of penetrating extra-thoracic injury, it must be performed in patients presenting pulseless with signs of life – pulseless electrical activity (PEA) or sudden cardiac arrest (SCA) in hospital or imminence of SCA (profound refractory shock). It must be remembered to avoid in patients with isolated cranial injuries [1].

M. F. Jucá Moscardi (✉)
University of Miami, Ryder Trauma Center, Miami, FL, USA

L. F. S. Brunello
Iwan Collaço Trauma Research Group, Hospital do Trabalhador Trauma Center, Federal University of Parana, Curitiba, Brazil

F. Saavedra Tomasich
Department of Surgery, Iwan Collaço Trauma Research Group, Hospital do Trabalhador Trauma Center, Federal University of Parana, Curitiba, Brazil

G. D. Pust
Division of Trauma and Surgical Critical Care, The DeWitt Daughtry Family Department of Surgery, Ryder Trauma Center/Jackson Memorial Hospital, Miller School of Medicine, University of Miami, Miami, FL, USA

© Springer Nature Switzerland AG 2020
A. Nasr et al. (eds.), *The Trauma Golden Hour*,
https://doi.org/10.1007/978-3-030-26443-7_9

The indication after blunt injury is to perform in patients presenting pulseless with signs of life – pulseless electrical activity (PEA) or sudden cardiac arrest (SCA) in hospital or imminence of SCA (profound refractory shock). It must be remembered to avoid in patients without signs of life and patients with isolated cranial injuries [1].

The best timing of closed-chest CPR plausible to start the thoracotomy is 15 minutes for penetrating traumas and 10 minutes for blunt traumas, and it can be performed in three different ways: (1) left anterolateral thoracotomy, (2) bilateral thoracotomy ("clamshell" incision), or (3) sternotomy; in which left anterolateral thoracotomy is preferred for EDT for its rapid access with simple instruments, the ability to perform on a patient with supine position, and easy "clamshell" incision converting, if needed [1, 3].

The possible maneuvers when performing an EDT are as follows: A. open the pericardium (if cardiac tamponade); B. repair the heart (if cardiac injury); C. control any thoracic hemorrhage; D. hilar cross-clamp (if air embolism); E. aortic cross-clamp (if extra thoracic hemorrhages); and F. internal heart massage [1, 3].

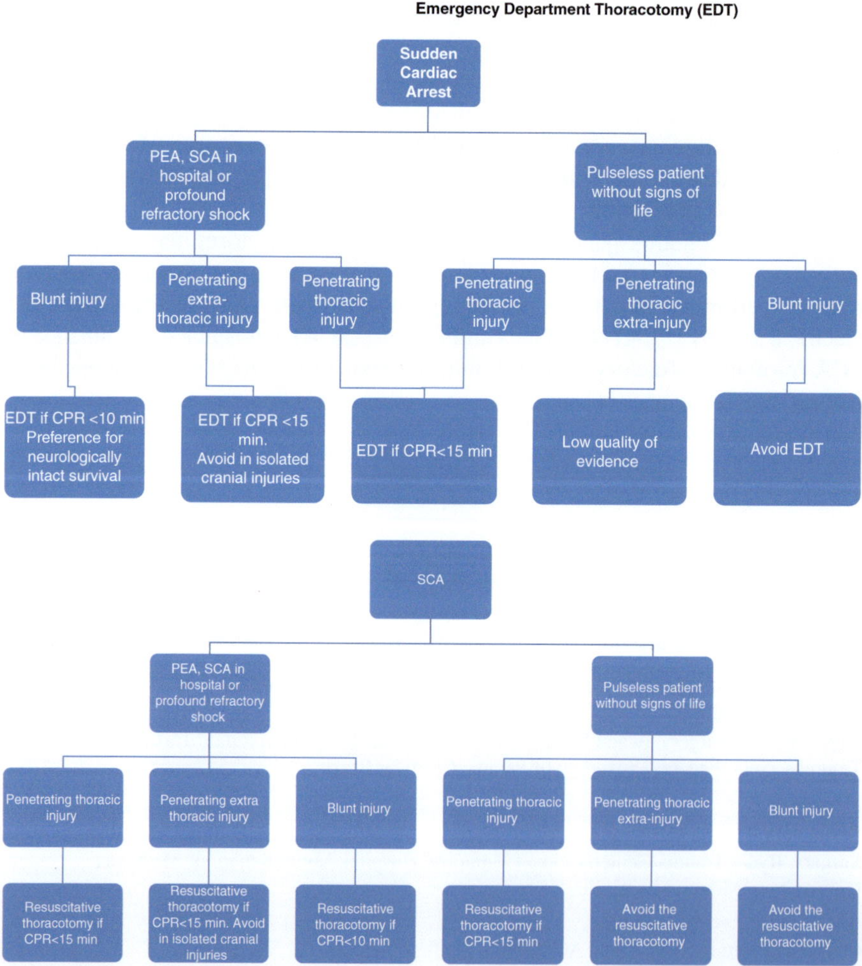

References

1. Seamon MJ, Haut ER, Van Arendonk K, Barbosa RR, Chiu WC, Dente CJ, et al. An evidence-based approach to patient selection for emergency department thoracotomy: a practice management guideline from the Eastern Association for the Surgery of Trauma. J Trauma Acute Care Surg. 2015;79(1):159–73.
2. American College of Surgeons. Advanced Trauma Life Support® (ATLS®): the tenth edition. Chicago, IL: American College of Surgeons (ACS), Committee on Trauma (COT); 2018. 377 p.
3. Mattox K, Moore EE, Feliciano D V. Trauma. 8th ed. New York: McGraw-Hill; 2017.

Traumatic Brain Injury

10

César Vinícius Grande, Leonardo Lasari Melo, Mariana F. Jucá Moscardi, and Antonio Marttos

10.1 Introduction

A head trauma is any injury that results in trauma to the skull, scalp, or brain. It has a great impact on general population's health, with a notable importance in both morbidity and mortality.

The main mechanism of traumatic brain injury (TBI) can be classified as a focal brain injury, a direct local trauma leading to concussion, laceration, and intracranial hemorrhage; or a diffuse brain injury, an acceleration/deceleration mechanism leading to diffuse axonal injury and cerebral edema. The outcome of a brain injury occurs in two different stages: primary lesion (occurs at the time of trauma) and secondary lesion (late clinical manifestations of a process started at the time of trauma).

Every patient with a suspected head trauma should initially undergo a focused neurological examination which consists of the Glasgow Coma Scale Score (GCS) (Table 10.1) plus pupillary reactivity that classifies the traumatic brain injury (TBI)

C. V. Grande
Department of Surgery, Hospital do Trabalhador Trauma Center,
Federal University of Parana, Curitiba, Brazil

L. L. Melo
Iwan Collaço Trauma Research Group, Department of Surgery, Hospital do Trabalhador
Trauma Center, Federal University of Parana, Curitiba, Brazil

M. F. Jucá Moscardi (✉)
University of Miami, Ryder Trauma Center, Miami, FL, USA

A. Marttos
William Lehman Injury Research Center, Division of Trauma & Surgical Critical Care,
Dewitt Daughtry Department of Surgery, Leonard M. Miller School of Medicine Miami,
University of Miami, Miami, FL, USA

© Springer Nature Switzerland AG 2020
A. Nasr et al. (eds.), *The Trauma Golden Hour*,
https://doi.org/10.1007/978-3-030-26443-7_10

Table 10.1 Glasgow Coma Scale

Behavior	Response	Score
Eye opening response	Spontaneously	4
	To speech	3
	To pain	2
	No response	1
Best verbal response	Oriented to time, place, and person	5
	Confused	4
	Inappropriate words	3
	Incomprehensible sounds	2
	No response	1
Best motor response	Obeys commands	6
	Moves to localized pain	5
	Flexion withdrawal from pain	4
	Abnormal flexion (decorticate)	3
	Abnormal extension (decerebrate)	2
	No response	1
Total score	*Best response*	15
	Comatose client	8 or less
	Totally unresponsive	3

as mild, moderate, or severe. It is very important to have information about the mechanism and time of trauma as well as the presence of symptoms such as nausea, vomiting, headache, loss or lowering of consciousness, behavior changes, seizures, diplopia, or irritability in children.

Some morphological aspects of the lesions are clear at the time of the first assessment. However, intracranial lesions are accurately diagnosed by computed tomography; and can be classified as focal (epidural hematomas, subdural hematomas, multiple or isolated intracerebral contusions) or diffuse (subarachnoid hemorrhage and diffuse axonal lesion).

Approximately 80% of the patients with traumatic brain injury are classified as mild, are usually alert or not symptomatic, and evolve to full recovery. Mild TBI is defined as GCS 14 or 15. These patients usually have a low risk to develop intracranial injury and are treated with symptomatics, home observation according to an informative protocol, hospital observation, or hospitalization depending on clinical presentation.

In victims of a moderate (GCS between 9 and 13) and a severe (GCS equal or lower than 8) TBI, it should be prioritized respiratory and hemodynamic conditions, cervical control, and the involvement of other surgical specialties in this patient care to determine the presence or nature of the associated lesions in other organs and systems.

In moderate TBI, patients are very symptomatic, presenting headache, frequent vomiting, occasional seizures, signs of basilar skull fracture, intoxication by alcohol or drugs, and children can be agitated and crying persistently. Moderate TBI corresponds to 10% of the cases; the conduct requires performing the trauma ABCDE assessment, hospitalization, skull and cervical spine computed tomography, and neurological and radiological sequential examination.

Victims of severe TBI (GCS less than 9) correspond to 10% of the cases and must be submitted to a secure airway and hemodynamic stabilization. In these patients, it is recommended to not postpone procedures and initial management to perform imagining exams, and to proceed with the ABCDE of the advanced life support, because usually, these patients present an associated hypotension due to the trauma mechanism. The hypotension should be corrected with volume replacement and adequate ventilation in order to minimize any secondary neurologic damage. After stabilization of the clinical and neurological conditions and multidisciplinary evaluation of trauma, the patient can be referred to imaging and other laboratory tests as diagnostic methods. Classical signs such as periorbital ecchymosis, mastoid ecchymosis (Battle's sign), hemodynamic or laceration of the external auditory canal, injury to the cranial nerves (I, II, VI, VII, or VIII pairs), rhinorrhea or otorrhea of cerebrospinal fluid, and multiple face fractures are suggestive of a basilar skull fracture. In these cases, there is also an emergency need for cranial tomography and these conditions can raise the graduation of the TBI to severe, even in conscious patients. Clinical approach in severe TBI requires infusion of saline solution or intravenous lactated Ringer, mannitol in the case of anisocoria, anticonvulsants, antiemetics, intravenous sedation, muscle relaxant, oral or nasotracheal intubation, mechanical ventilation, and ICU. Surgical approach of TBI involves wound sutures, treating cranial sags, identifying and treating gunshot and stab wounds, drainage of hematomas, interposition of ventricular or intraparenchymal catheters for intracranial pressure measurement, and decompressive craniotomies to relieve refractory or acute hypertension by diffuse swelling.

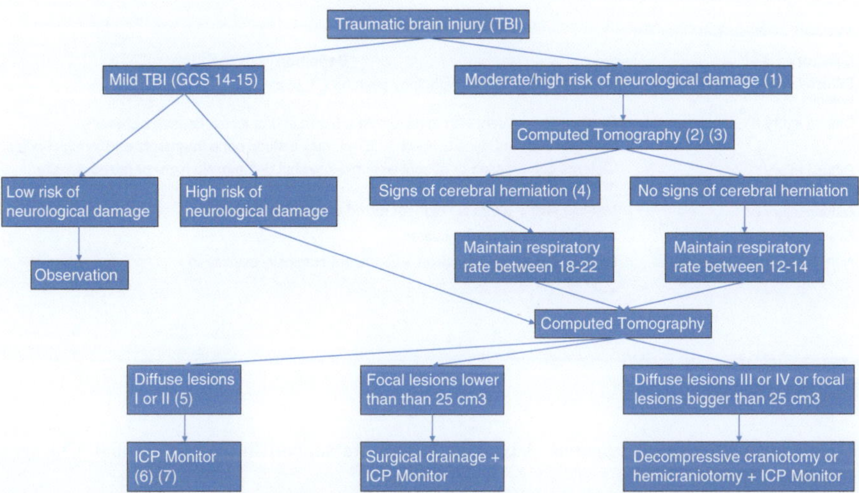

10.2 Conclusion

(1) Change in the level of consciousness, loss of consciousness, seizure, severe headache, lacunar amnesia, nausea or vomiting, age greater than 60 years and less than 2 years, cranial fracture, signs of basilar skull fracture, otorrhagia.

(2) Secure airway + cervical immobilization; O_2 + oximeter; volume replacement. Intubation with FiO_2 of 100%, volume of 6–8 ml/min and PEEP of 5 mmHg. Orogastric tube, bladder catheter, and rectal examination.

(3) Intracranial hypertension:
   - If blood pressure is normal: mannitol 20%
   - If low blood pressure: 20% NaCl
     - If systolic blood pressure lower than 90 mmHg: consider blood transfusion and initiate vasoactive drug

(4) Signs of cerebral herniation are anisocoria, abnormal motor posture, neurogenic hyperpnea, and ataxic respiration pattern.

(5) Diffuse lesions type I associated with two of the following factors: hypotension, over 40 years old, abnormal motor posture; or diffuse lesions type II. In case of no visible CT lesion and no risk factor, the patient should stay in observation.

(6) Intracranial pressure, external ventricular shunt, transcranial doppler, cerebral tissue oxygen pressure, continuous electroencephalogram.

(7) The monitoring of the intracranial pressure is appropriate in patients with severe TBI and with altered CT at admission (bruising, contusion, edema, or compression of the basal cisterns). It is also indicated in patients with severe TBI in the presence of two or more risk factors: age greater than 40 years, single or bilateral pathological motor posture, and systolic blood pressure lower than 90 mmHg.

(8) Marshall Tomographic Classification for patients with GCS lower than 9.

Marshall CT classification of TBI

Category	Definition
Diffuse injury I (no visible pathology)	No visible intra-cranial pathology seen on CT scan
Diffuse injury II	Cisterns are present with midline shift < 5 mm and/or lesion densities present
	No high- or mixed-density lesion > 25 ml, may include bone fragments and foreign bodies
Diffuse injury III	Cisterns compressed or absent with mid-line shift 0–5 mm No high- or mixed-density lesion > 25 ml
Diffuse injury IV	Mid-line shift > 5 mm No high- or mixed-density lesion > 25 ml
Evacuated mass lesion	Any lesion surgically evacuated
Non-evacuated mass lesion	High- or mixed-density lesion > 25 ml, not surgically evacuated

Bibliography

1. American College of Surgeons. Advanced trauma life support instructors manual. Chicago; 2004.
2. Greenberg MS. Manual de Neurocirurgia 5°. Ed.

3. Timmons, S.D. Current trends in neurotrauma care. Crit Care Med, 2010;38(9 Suppl):S431–44. https://doi.org/10.1097/CCM.0b013e3181ec57ab.
4. Bullock R, Chesnut R, Clifton G, et al. Guidelines for the management of severe head injury. New York: Brain Trauma Foundation; 1996.
5. Andrade AF, Ciquini O Jr, Figueiredo EG, Brock RS, Marino R Jr. Diretrizes do atendimento ao paciente com traumatismo cranioencefálico. Arquivos Brasileiros de Neurocirurgia. Sociedade Brasileira de Neurocirurgia, São Paulo, v.18, n.3, p.131–176, set.1999.
6. Fluxograma para diretrizes de atendimento inicial ao paciente politraumatizado com TCE grave. 2009. Disponível em http://www.neurotraumabrasil.org.
7. Chesnut RM. Avoidance of hypotension: conditio sine qua non of successful severe head-injury management. J Trauma. 1997;42:S4–9.

Penetrating Neck Trauma

Mariana F. Jucá Moscardi, Silvania Klug Pimentel,
Fernanda Cristina Silva, Jean Raitz Novais,
and Antonio Marttos

11.1 Introduction

The trauma of the cervical region is characterized by its high complexity and high morbidity. There is no other segment in the body that contains structures representative of so many systems in a space as confined as the neck: respiratory, digestive, vascular, central and peripheral, lymphatic, and endocrine systems. Cervical trauma can be divided into penetrating – lesions that extend beyond the platysma muscle – and not penetrating.

This chapter is dedicated only to penetrating cervical trauma, which requires special investigation due to the presence of important aerodigestive and neurovascular structures located below the platysma muscle.

The penetrative cervical trauma approach has changed substantially over the past decades, from mandatory surgical exploration to conservative treatment. The initial management is decisive in the success of the patient's treatment. Mortality from

M. F. Jucá Moscardi (✉)
University of Miami, Ryder Trauma Center, Miami, FL, USA

S. K. Pimentel · F. C. Silva
Department of Surgery, Hospital do Trabalhador Trauma Center,
Federal University of Parana, Curitiba, Brazil

J. R. Novais
Iwan Collaço Trauma Research Group, Department of Surgery, Hospital do Trabalhador
Trauma Center, Federal University of Parana, Curitiba, Brazil

A. Marttos
William Lehman Injury Research Center, Division of Trauma & Surgical Critical Care,
Dewitt Daughtry Department of Surgery, Leonard M. Miller School of Medicine Miami,
University of Miami, Miami, FL, USA

© Springer Nature Switzerland AG 2020
A. Nasr et al. (eds.), *The Trauma Golden Hour*,
https://doi.org/10.1007/978-3-030-26443-7_11

severe vascular lesions up to 50%, and late complications such as pseudoaneurysms and arteriovenous fistulas, which may affect long-term outcomes, should be considered. Therefore, the correct management, at the right time, is fundamental.

11.2 Zones of the Neck

The neck is divided into three zones anatomically delimited: Zone I, Zone II, and Zone III. The importance of evaluating the affected area is that it helps to predict the structures affected by trauma in each region, thus helping the management of the situation. Zone I extends between the clavicle and the cricoid cartilage; Zone II extends between cricoid cartilage and the angle of the mandible; Zone III extends between the angle of the mandible and the base of the skull. Figure 11.1 represents different neck zones.

11.3 Initial Evaluation

The initial evaluation of any trauma should always follow the ABC sequence of the trauma; in the cervical trauma, the same principle must be followed. The first step is to evaluate and manage the airway ensuring a safe airway. Early intubation must be considered in cases of hypoxemia, inability to ventilate, stridor, expanding hematoma, gross hemorrhage, or decreased loss of consciousness. Cricothyroidotomy should be considered before the airway is lost. In the absence of blunt trauma, C-Spine immobilization is rarely necessary.

Once the airway is secured, the neck should be fully evaluated. The location of the wounds should be evaluated to get a sense of the neck zone. The wound should be neither explored nor probed. If the wound does not penetrate the muscle

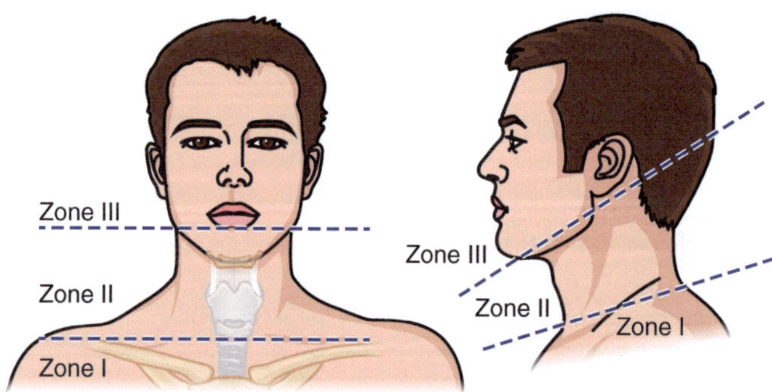

Fig. 11.1 Zones of the neck

platysma, no further evaluation is required. Any external hemorrhage should be managed by direct pressure. Patients should be evaluated for changes in phonation, odynophagia, cranial nerve abnormalities, paresthesia, or weakness in the extremities. An X-ray should be obtained (AP and lateral film) to evaluate the trajectory and ensure that there are no secondary fragments that might alter the approach. Insertion of an NG tube should wait until the patient is in the operating room or better evaluated with image exams.

11.4   Indications for Immediate Operation

There are cases where the patient should be taken immediately to the operating room because further evaluation with imaging tests would delay the therapeutic measure, risking the patient's life.

In some cases, the patient should be taken immediately to the operating room so as not to delay the therapeutic measures. Shock, active hemorrhage, expanding or pulsatile hematoma, airway compression or dyspnea, and air bubbling through wound and instrument in situ indicate that the patient should be taken immediately to the operating room, as the delay in initiating the therapeutic measures can be fatal.

11.5   Patients with No Immediate Criteria for Operation

In cases in which there are no indications of immediate exploratory cervicotomy, we must separate the ducts according to the affected cervical zone. Given the challenges with surgical exposure, traumas in Zones I and III should be evaluated mainly through CT angiography. Injuries in Zone I should be evaluated for esophagus or airway problems if the patient has symptoms that suggest it (odynophagia, hematemesis, subcutaneous emphysema, and hoarseness). Injuries in Zone I might require cardiac, thoracic, or vascular surgery. Injuries in Zone III might require expertise from ENT (for those involving the hypopharynx) or vascular/neurosurgery to address injuries to the high internal carotid artery. Zone II traumas require CT angiogram to evaluate the carotid and vertebral arteries. If the patient has odynophagia, hematemesis, or if the CT suggests that the trajectory is close to the esophagus, contrast esophagography or esophagoscopy should be performed. Evaluation of the larynx and airway is indicated if there is subcutaneous emphysema, hemoptysis, and hoarseness, or the trajectory is close to the airway. This is usually performed by laryngoscopy or bronchoscopy, depending on the level of injury. Instead of imaging exams, it is possible to indicate surgical exploration with an incision along the anterior sternomastoid. This requires evaluation of the vessels, the esophagus, and the larynx/trachea. The trajectory of the wound should be followed.

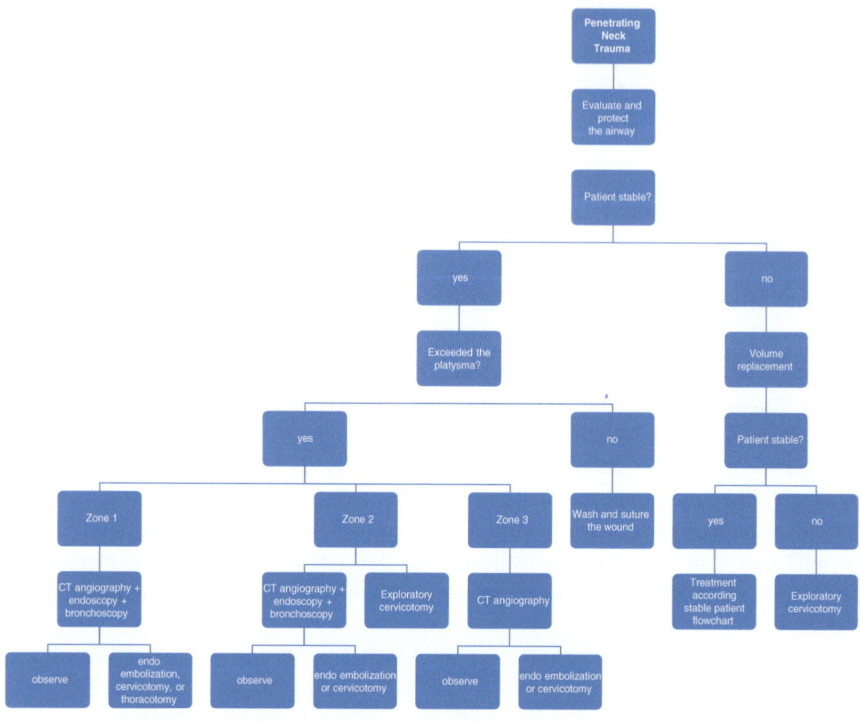

Bibliography

1. Cassimiro AD, et al. Abordagem do Trauma Cervical Penetrante na zona II. Rev Med Minas Gerais. 2010;20(4 Suppl 2):S1–S147.
2. Britt LD, Weireter LJ, Cole JF. Management of acute neck injuries. In: Mattox KL, Feliciano DV, Moore EE. Trauma. 6ª ed. New York: McGraw-Hill; 2007.
3. David BH, Maisel RH. Penetrating and blunt trauma of the neck. Cummings otolaryngology – head and neck surgery. 5th ed. Philadelphia, PA: Mosby; 2010. p. 1625–35.

Blunt Cervical Trauma

12

Seung Hoon Shin, Mariana F. Jucá Moscardi,
Thamyle Moda de S. Rezende, João Ricardo Martinelli,
and Rishi Rattan

While incidence of cervical spine injury is relatively rare at 1–6.2% [1] with unstable injuries requiring intervention being even rare, missed injury or delayed treatment may result in long-term disability and life-threatening complications.

In particular, lesions above C7 can lead to respiratory distress or failure due to loss of central innervation of the phrenic nerves, and lesions above T6 can lead to neurogenic shock from loss of vasomotor tone and sympathetic innervation to the heart.

Cervical spine immobilization during prehospital transport varies according to local practice, with limited data not yet resulting in clear recommendations on whether or not the cervical spine needs to be routinely immobilized. Practice should be guided by multidisciplinary local protocols.

Strict immobilization should be maintained, including during head and neck maneuvers, such as obtaining an airway or placement of a central venous catheter, until the cervical spine is cleared. Cervical collars should be removed as soon as safely possible because continued use of the c-collar has risks of pressure ulcers,

S. H. Shin
Ryder Trauma Center – Jackson Health System, Miami, FL, USA

Miller School of Medicine, University of Miami, Miami, FL, USA

M. F. Jucá Moscardi (✉)
University of Miami, Ryder Trauma Center, Miami, FL, USA

T. M. de S. Rezende · J. R. Martinelli
Iwan Collaço Trauma Research Group, Department of Surgery, Hospital do Trabalhador
Trauma Center, Federal University of Parana, Curitiba, Brazil

R. Rattan
Division of Trauma Surgery & Critical Care, DeWitt Daughtry Family Department of
Surgery, Miller School of Medicine, University of Miami, Miami, FL, USA

© Springer Nature Switzerland AG 2020
A. Nasr et al. (eds.), *The Trauma Golden Hour*,
https://doi.org/10.1007/978-3-030-26443-7_12

decreased cerebral venous return, increased intracranial pressure and secondary brain injury, and difficulties with airway and central line management.

The Canadian Cervical spine Rule (CCR) is a clinical assessment tool to guide clinical decision-making around using imaging to clear the cervical spine. Multiple studies have shown that CCR has superior sensitivity (99.4 vs 90.7%), specificity (45.1 vs 36.8%), and negative predictive value (100 vs 99.4%) to other guidelines, such as the National Emergency X-Radiography Utilization Study (NEXUS) Low-Risk Criteria [2].

For the patients who cannot be cleared clinically by CCR, computed tomography (CT) scan will be the first-line diagnostic modality. When an adequate scan is performed, with at least 3 mm cuts using at least a 16-slice multidetector device, the false-negative rate was 0.03%. Of note, however, all patients had a neurological deficit on physical exam. In patients with suspected cervical spine injury and no neurological deficit on physical exam, the false-negative rate for adequate CT scan was 0% [3]. However, the most recent Eastern Association for the Surgery of Trauma guidelines recommend removal of the cervical collar in even obtunded patients with a negative but adequately performed CT scan, which suggests that physical exam findings are not relevant. Importantly, the recommendation is based on low-quality evidence, resulting in a weak or conditional recommendation, and with the caveat that there may be a non-zero rate of missed cervical spine injuries, though these are very unlikely to result in surgical intervention or permanent disability, and discovery of injury on MRI after a negative CT rarely changes management [4–6]. Thus, in patients with a neurological deficit and a normal CT scan, magnetic resonance imaging (MRI) should be considered. Consultation with a spine specialist may be warranted in these scenarios.

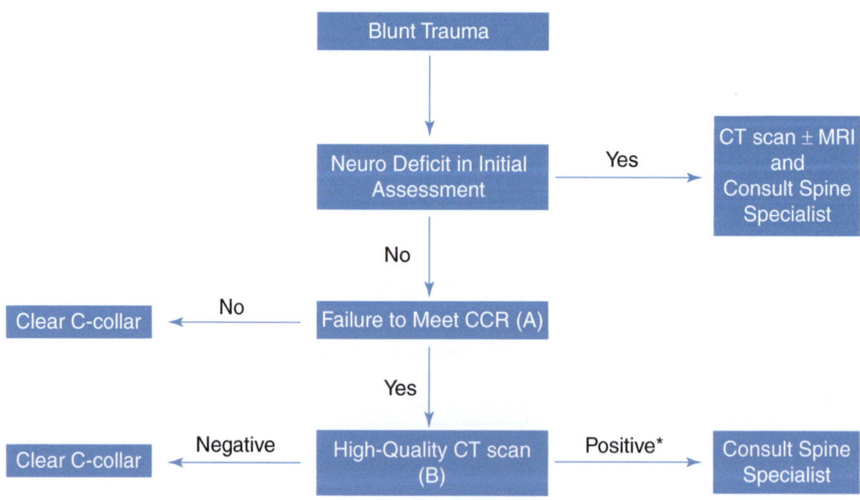

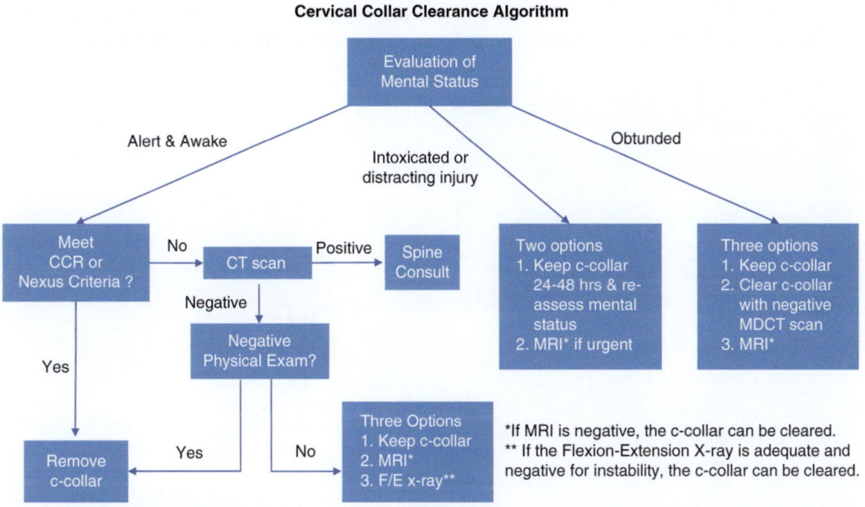

12.1 Conclusion

A. CCR is based on three high-risk criteria, five low-risk criteria, and the ability of patients to rotate their necks (see Fig. 12.1). If a patient meets all the criteria and is able to rotate his/her neck, the c-collar can be cleared.

B. High-quality CT scan refers axial thickness of less than 3 mm.

  ∗ Most common positive CT scan findings are fractures of transverse process (TP) and/or spinous process (SP) fractures. Isolated transverse or spinous process fractures and negative for ligament injury in CT scan and the patient is GCS 15 and there is no midline tenderness or neurologic deficit, the c-collar could be safely removed [7].

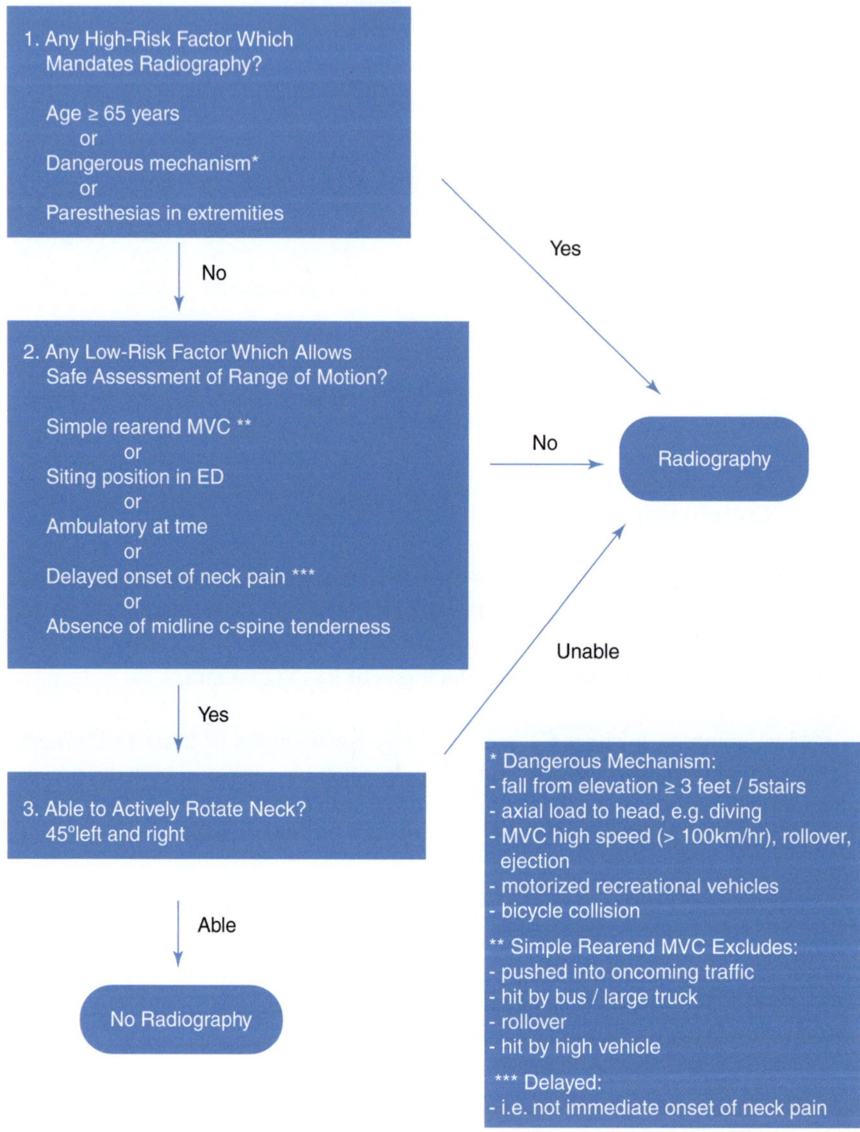

Fig. 12.1 Adult Canadian C-spine Rule [2]

References

1. Young AJ, Wolfe L, Tinkoff G, et al. Assessing incidence and risk factors of cervical spine injury in blunt trauma patients using the National Trauma Data Bank. Am Surg. 2015;81(9):879–83.
2. Stiell IG, Clement CM, McKnight RD, et al. The Canadian C-spine rule versus the NEXUS low-risk criteria in patients with trauma. N Engl J Med. 2003;349(26):2510–8.
3. Inaba K, Byerly S, Bush LD, et al. Cervical spinal clearance: a prospective Western Trauma Association Multi-institutional Trial. J Trauma Acute Care Surg. 2016;81(6):1122–30.
4. Como JJ, et al. Practice management guidelines for identification of cervical spine injuries following trauma: update from the eastern association for the surgery of trauma practice management guidelines committee. J Trauma. 2009;67(3):651–9.
5. Patel MB, Humble SS, Cullinane DC, et al. Cervical spine collar clearance in the obtunded adult blunt trauma patient: a systematic review and practice management guideline from the Eastern Association for the Surgery of Trauma. J Trauma Acute Care Surg. 2015;78(2):430–41.
6. Resnick S, Inaba K, Karamanos E, et al. Clinical relevance of magnetic resonance imaging in cervical spine clearance: a prospective study. JAMA Surg. 2014;149(9):934–9.
7. Duane TM, Young AJ, Vanguri P. Defining the cervical spine clearance algorithm: a single-institution prospective study of more than 9,000 patients. J Trauma Acute Care Surg. 2016;81(3):541–7.

Spinal Cord Injury

13

Xavier Soler Graells, Marcel Luiz Benato,
Pedro Grein del Santoro, Haiana Lopes Cavalheiro,
Mariana F. Jucá Moscardi, Marcelo Tsuyoshi Yamane,
Andrea Rachel Marcadis, and Antonio Marttos

13.1 Introduction

Spinal cord injury (SCI) occurs predominantly in young adult males. The thoracic spine and lumbar spine are the most frequent sites of fracture of the axial skeleton and account for about 89% of spine fractures. Of thoracolumbar fractures, two-thirds occur in the thoracolumbar transition between T11 and L2. Most (50%) of the thoracic fractures occur at T12, and most (60%) lumbar fractures occur at L1. It is important to note that 10–15% of all patients with severe head trauma have associated lesions in the cervical spine, and therefore, the presence of SCI must be assumed in all polytrauma patients until proven otherwise. For this reason, the cervical collar should be placed in all polytrauma patients until SCI is ruled out. Once an SCI is ruled out, the long spine board should be removed as soon as possible in order to avoid pressure ulcers.

X. S. Graells · M. L. Benato · P. G. del Santoro
Department of Surgery, Hospital do Trabalhador Trauma Center, Federal University of Parana, Curitiba, Brazil

H. L. Cavalheiro · M. T. Yamane
Iwan Collaço Trauma Research Group, Department of Surgery, Hospital do Trabalhador Trauma Center, Federal University of Parana, Curitiba, Brazil

M. F. Jucá Moscardi (✉)
University of Miami, Ryder Trauma Center, Miami, FL, USA

A. R. Marcadis
Department of Surgery, University of Miami, Miller School of Medicine, Jackson Memorial Hospital, Miami, FL, USA

A. Marttos
William Lehman Injury Research Center, Division of Trauma & Surgical Critical Care, Dewitt Daughtry Department of Surgery, Leonard M. Miller School of Medicine Miami, University of Miami, Miami, FL, USA

© Springer Nature Switzerland AG 2020
A. Nasr et al. (eds.), *The Trauma Golden Hour*,
https://doi.org/10.1007/978-3-030-26443-7_13

On neurological examination of a potential SCI patient, one should pay attention to cranial nerve abnormalities that suggest lesions at the occipito-cervical junction, C5-T1, and L2-S1. Tingling or paralysis of a limb suggests severe injury to the spinal cord. Rectal examination is an essential part of the neurological examination and should assess anal sphincter tone, anal and perianal sensitivity, and anal and bulbocavernosus reflexes. In contrast to spinal shock which is a transient reflex depression of cord function below the level of injury, neurogenic shock is characterized by hypotension and bradycardia resulting from the loss of vasomotor tone and sympathetic innervation to the heart. In addition to the neurological examination, the diagnostic workup includes radiographs, computed tomography, and magnetic resonance imaging for visualization of soft-tissue lesions.

Once SCI has been diagnosed, it can be further characterized based on injury patterns. Paraplegia and quadriplegia from SCI can be either complete or incomplete. If there is any motor or sensory function below the level of injury, it is considered an incomplete lesion. There are also characteristic patterns of neurological injury that are defined spinal cord syndromes, such as central cord syndrome, anterior cord syndrome, and Brown-Séquard syndrome.

Central cord syndrome is characterized by a disproportionately greater loss of motor strength in the upper extremities compared to the lower extremities, and is associated with bladder dysfunction and varying degrees of sensory loss below the level of the lesion. It most commonly occurs after neck hyperextension in patients with preexisting cervical spondylosis. The mechanism of injury is usually a forward fall resulting in neck hyperextension and facial impact. The prognosis for a patient with central cord syndrome is better than that of other incomplete lesions.

The anterior cord syndrome is characterized by injury to the anterior two-thirds of the spinal cord, compromising the motor and sensory pathways. Patients generally present with paraplegia and bilateral loss of temperature and pain sensation. With this syndrome, the dorsal columns, and therefore fine touch and proprioception, remain intact. Anterior cord syndrome has the worst prognosis of all incomplete lesions and usually occurs due to ischemia from injury to the anterior spinal artery.

Brown-Séquard syndrome results from cord hemisection, usually caused by penetrating trauma. It is characterized by ipsilateral loss of motor and position sense at the level of the lesion, with contralateral loss of pain and temperature sensation one to two levels below the level of the lesion.

Oftentimes, fractures of the cervical spine with subluxation are amenable to closed reduction. This treatment consists of a longitudinal traction using skull tongs. Closed reduction generally avoids surgery and promotes neurological improvement in some cases. In a study of 82 patients with cervical subluxation, this procedure was successfully performed in 98% of patients, and the average time to achieve the reduction was 2 hours. Sometimes, however, operative management is required for stabilization of the spine or reduction of dislocations and decompression of neural elements. Indications for operative management of cervical spine injuries include significant spinal cord compression with neurological deficits that do not respond to closed reduction, or an unstable vertebral fracture or dislocation. Most penetrating injuries require surgical exploration to remove foreign bodies and wash out the wound.

Regarding the use of steroids in SCI, there is still debate among professionals, although recent studies have demonstrated the lack of efficacy of high-dose methylprednisolone in the acute treatment of patients with spinal cord injuries. The corticosteroid randomization after significant head injury (CRASH) trial randomized over 10,000 adults with head injury and Glasgow Coma Scale (GCS) 14 or less to receive corticosteroid (methylprednisolone) or placebo and showed an increase in mortality in the steroid group compared to the placebo group. However, in specific injuries such as spinal contusions or traumatic central cord syndrome, steroid administration may still be warranted. The therapeutic approach to spinal cord injuries should be multidisciplinary, and include physical and occupational therapy in order to give the patient the best possible chance of recovery from such an injury.

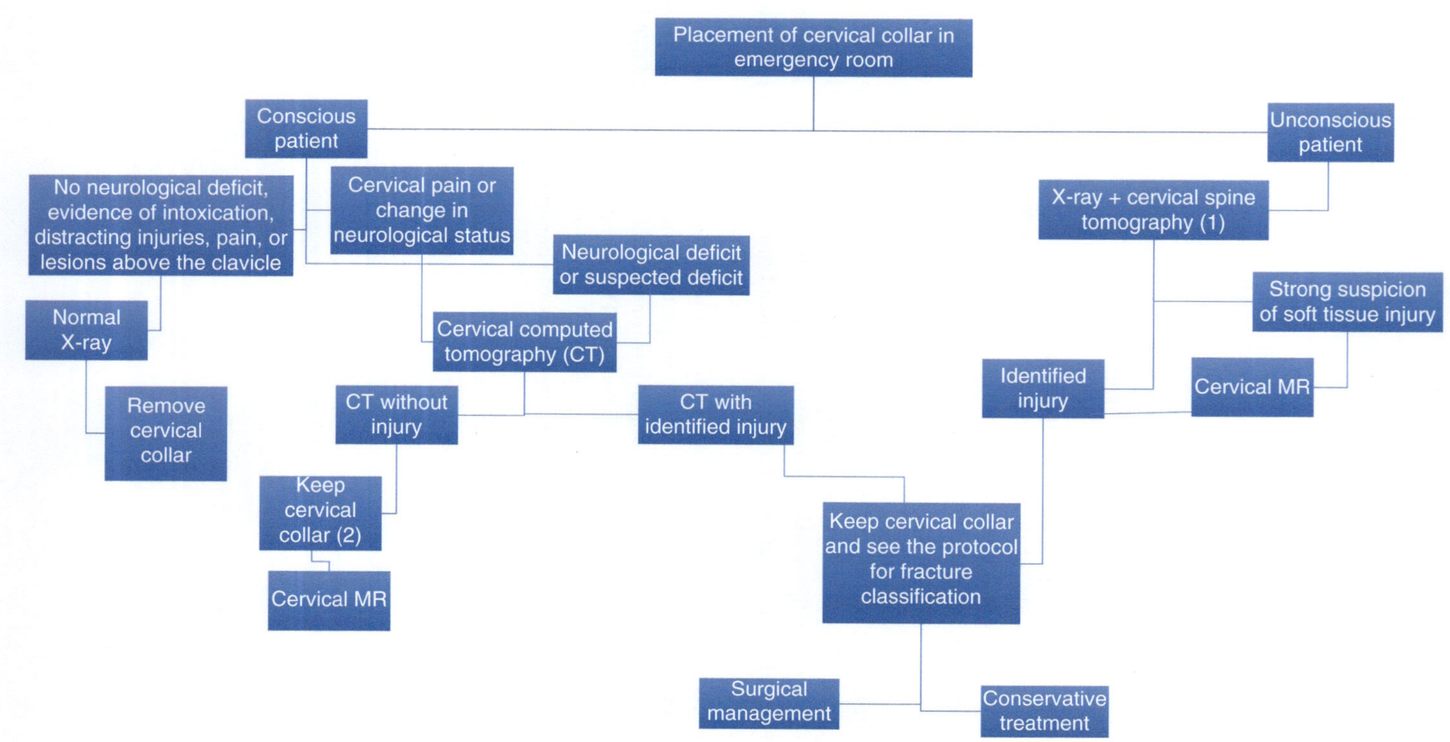

Placement of cervical collar in emergency room
Conscious patient
Unconscious patient
No neurological deficit, evidence of intoxication, distracting injuries, pain, or lesions above the clavicle
Cervical pain or change in neurological status
X-ray + cervical spine tomography (1)
Neurological deficit or suspected deficit
Strong suspicion of soft tissue injury
Normal X-ray
Cervical computed tomography (CT)
Identified injury
Cervical MR
Remove cervical collar
CT without injury
CT with identified injury
Keep cervical collar (2)
Keep cervical collar and see the protocol for fracture classification
Cervical MR
Surgical management
Conservative treatment

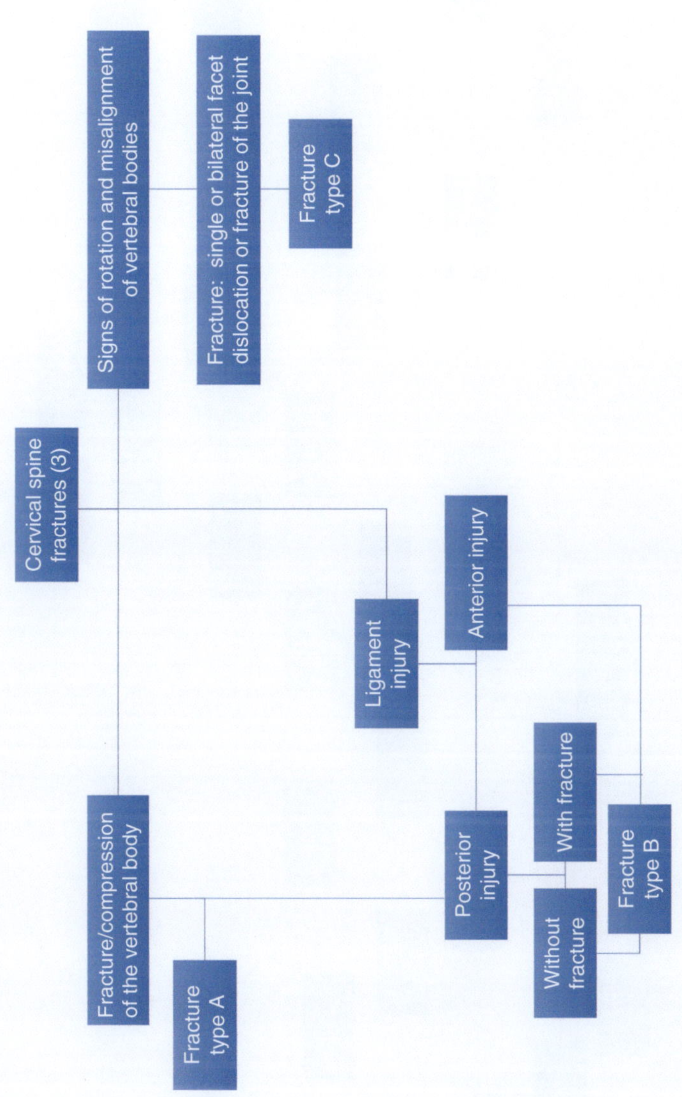
Cervical spine fractures (3)
Signs of rotation and misalignment of vertebral bodies
Fracture: single or bilateral facet dislocation or fracture of the joint
Fracture type C
Fracture/compression of the vertebral body
Fracture type A
Ligament injury
Anterior injury
Posterior injury
With fracture
Without fracture
Fracture type B

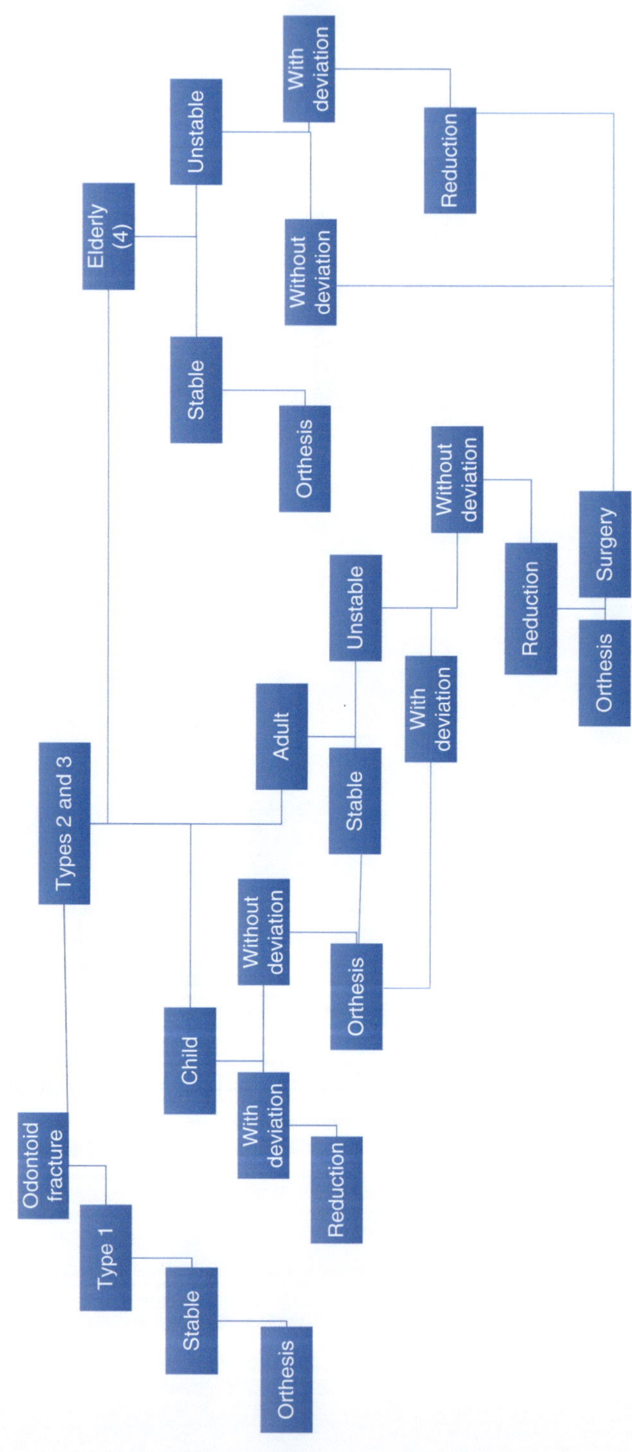
Odontoid fracture
Type 1
Stable
Orthesis
Types 2 and 3
Child
Adult
Elderly (4)
With deviation
Reduction
Without deviation
Orthesis
Stable
Unstable
With deviation
Without deviation
Reduction
Surgery
Orthesis
Stable
Orthesis
Unstable
With deviation
Without deviation
Reduction

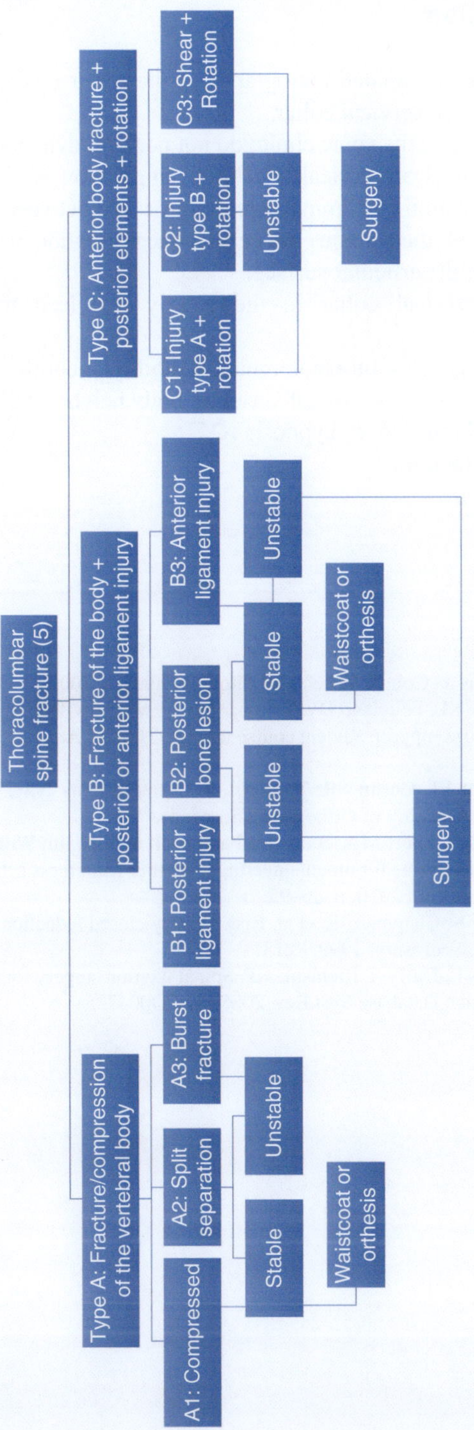

Thoracolumbar spine fracture (5)
Type A: Fracture/compression of the vertebral body
Type B: Fracture of the body + posterior or anterior ligament injury
Type C: Anterior body fracture + posterior elements + rotation
A1: Compressed
A2: Split separation
A3: Burst fracture
B1: Posterior ligament injury
B2: Posterior bone lesion
B3: Anterior ligament injury
C1: Injury type A + rotation
C2: Injury type B + rotation
C3: Shear + Rotation
Stable
Unstable
Waistcoat or orthesis
Surgery

13.2 Conclusion

(1) If the X-ray and computed tomography of the cervical spine do not show any lesion, remove the cervical collar.
(2) Refer the patient to the spine clinic; do not perform dynamic X-ray.
(3) Radiological signs of cervical instability: angulation >11° between vertebral bodies, translocation >3.5 mm, increased distance between spinous processes, misalignment of the spinous processes, facet rotation in profile incidence, enlargement of the articular surface.
(4) Use of the cervical collar in the elderly can lead to myelopathy and pseudarthrosis.
(5) Radiological signs of thoracolumbar instability: neurological deficit, spinal cord compression >50%, loss of vertebral body height > 50%, contiguous fractures, vertebral translation, kyphosis >25°.
(6) Osteoporosis fracture.
(7) Chance's fracture.

Bibliography

1. Lesões Traumáticas da Coluna Vertebral; Editora Bevilacqua 2005.
2. Moore EE, Mattox KL, Feliciano DV. Trauma. 8th ed. McGraw-Hill; 2017.
3. Advanced trauma life support: student course manual. 10th ed. American College of Surgeons; 2017.
4. Zigler JE, Eismont FJ, Garfin SR, Vaccaro AR. Spine trauma AAOS. 2nd ed. Rosemont, Illinois: American Academy of Orthopaedic Surgeons.
5. Stahel PF, Heyde CE, Flierl MA, et al. Head and neck injuries. In: Wilkerson JA, Moore EE, Zafren K, editors. Medicine for mountaineering and other wilderness activities. 6th ed. Seattle: The Mountaineers Books; 2010. p. 86–95.
6. Grant GA, Mirza SK, Chapman JR, et al. Risk of early closed reduction in cervical spine subluxation injuries. J Neurosurg. 1999;90:13.
7. Bagnall AM, Jones L, Duffy S, Riemsma RP. Spinal fixation surgery for acute traumatic spinal cord injury. Cochrane Database Syst Rev. 2008;(1):CD004725.

Blunt Thoracic Trauma

14

Nelson Thomé Zardo, Eduardo Lopes Martins,
Gassan Traya, Mariana F. Jucá Moscardi,
and Antonio Marttos

14.1 Introduction

In the modern management of trauma, the conducts in thoracic lesions depend on the trauma mechanism (penetrating × blunt), on the severity (stable × instable), and on the lesion site (wall × pleura × lungs). Severe thoracic trauma requires a fast diagnosis and treatment; there is no time for imaging exams with high accuracy and elaborate diagnosis. The initial management of these patients is guided by ATLS. The priorities are to secure an airway, adequate ventilation with oxygen supply, and treatment of shock. The thorax is right in the primary survey of trauma in the ABC of ATLS. The evaluation of the suboptimal chest X-ray obtained in the emergency room should be considered as an extension of the ABC of ATLS regarding thoracic trauma.

In the secondary physical examination, the total surface of the chest should be inspected to verify if there are any wounds, lacerations, and contusions. Rather than auscultating, the movement of the chest wall should be observed in some respiratory cycles, searching for paradoxical movements or any evident deformity. The

N. T. Zardo
Iwan Collaço Trauma Research Group, Department of Surgery, Hospital do Trabalhador
Trauma Center, Federal University of Parana, Curitiba, Brazil

E. L. Martins · G. Traya
Department of Surgery, Hospital do Trabalhador Trauma Center,
Federal University of Parana, Curitiba, Brazil

M. F. Jucá Moscardi (✉)
University of Miami, Ryder Trauma Center, Miami, FL, USA

A. Marttos
William Lehman Injury Research Center, Division of Trauma & Surgical Critical Care,
Dewitt Daughtry Department of Surgery, Leonard M. Miller School of Medicine Miami,
University of Miami, Miami, FL, USA

© Springer Nature Switzerland AG 2020
A. Nasr et al. (eds.), *The Trauma Golden Hour*,
https://doi.org/10.1007/978-3-030-26443-7_14

palpation of the chest wall can reveal rib fractures, clavicle fractures, painful points, and subcutaneous emphysema. The evaluation of the pulses and measurement of the blood pressure in both arms could reveal lesions of the gathered thoracic vessels. Neurological evaluation is needed to search for lesions of the brachial plexus. Several evaluations should be done over time to identify progressive changes in the respiratory function, such as a small pneumothorax that increases in volume. Oximeter, arterial gasometry, and early chest X-ray are essential diagnostic methods and provide reliable parameters to indicate intubation and mechanical ventilation in patients with severe blunt thoracic trauma.

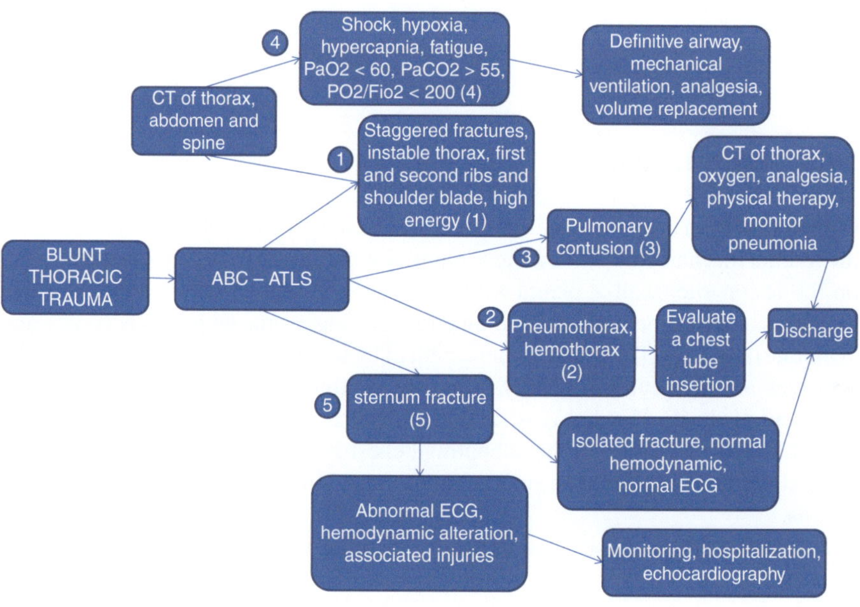

14.2 Conclusion

Rib fractures (10% of the patients), isolated or multiple, because of the pain, cause the restriction of the expansion of the thoracic wall, leading to an abnormal respiratory mechanics. However, most of the observed dysfunctions after a severe blunt thoracic trauma are secondary to the subjacent pulmonary contusion. Intrapleural damage is an uncommon result after fractures caused by antero-posterior compression of the chest. There is a higher chance of pleural lesion in fractures due to direct trauma to the chest. Special attention should be given to the fractures below the ninth rib because of its relation to injuries in the spleen and liver. Thoracic and abdominal lesions could happen even if there is no rib fracture, especially in children. In elderly, due to bone fragility, rib fractures usually happen without any other associated thoracic injury.

(1) Fractures of the first rib, second rib, and shoulder blade, and staggered rib fractures are related to high-energy trauma. Recognizing these injuries is important, as these require immediate care and search for thoracic, spine, great vessels, and abdominal lesions. Thoracic and abdominal CT can be used as supportive diagnostic method.

(2) After identifying a hemothorax or pneumothorax by X-ray, the placement of a chest tube should be discussed. In case of small pneumothorax in stable and asymptomatic patients without mechanical ventilation, there is a possibility to observe the patient for 12 hours and perform serial X-rays over time. In case of hemothorax identified by fluids in posterior costophrenic angles in the X-ray, which means a bleeding greater than 300 mL, should be placed a chest tube and be aware of the indications to a thoracotomy (immediate drainage of 1500 mL or drainage of 200 mL/hour for 4 hours). In small hemothorax, detected by CT and not by X-ray, in asymptomatic patients, we can proceed with observation of the patient, analgesia, and radiological control. It should be kept in mind that a doubt about the placement of a chest tube in a patient with a small hemopneumothorax should be considered as an encouraging factor.

 In an unstable thorax, there is a segment of the chest wall that moves in the opposite direction of the rest of the thoracic wall during spontaneous respiratory movements. This paradoxical movement is identified in the initial physical examination during inspection and observation of respiratory cycles.

(3) Due to high-energy direct trauma that causes unstable thorax, the severity of the subadjacent pulmonary lesion following alveolar bleeding has a greater role than the paradoxical movement in the impairment of lung function in gas exchange. The initial treatment consists of supplementary oxygenation, respiratory and motor physical therapy, analgesia, intercostal nerves blockage, aspiration of the superior airways, and continuous evaluation.

(4) The required aggressive volume replacement in polytraumatized patients results in clinical worsening of the pulmonary contusion and we should keep in mind that the indications of a definitive airway and mechanical ventilation depend on the objective evidence of respiratory failure manifested by the following criteria: clinical signs of fatigue, respiratory frequency greater than 35 or lower than 8 per minute, PaO_2 lower than 60 mmHg, $PaCO_2$ greater than 55 mmHg, PaO_2/FiO_2 ratio lower than 200, clinical evidence of shock, severe TBI, and severe associated surgical injuries.

(5) Sternum fracture results from a direct impact. When there is isolated sternum fracture, the chance of a myocardial injury is low; and if the patient is hemodynamically stable and without any radiological or electrocardiographic alteration, hospitalization is not required. Treatment consists of analgesics and rarely surgery is needed.

Bibliography

1. Moore EE, Mattox KL, Feliciano DV. Manual do Trauma. 4nd ed. Porto Alegre: Artmed; 2006.
2. Vieira HM Jr, Drumond DAF. Protocolos em Trauma. Rio de Janeiro: Medbook; 2009.
3. American College of Surgeons. Advanced trauma life support. 8th ed. Chicago, IL: American College of Surgeons; 2008.
4. Moore EE, Mattox KL, Feliciano DV. Trauma. 6th ed. McGraw-Hill Education; 2008.
5. McGillicuddy D, Rosen P. Diagnostic dilemmas and current controversies in blunt chest trauma. Emerg Med Clin North Am. 2007;25(3):695–711, viii–ix. Review.
6. Yadav K, Jalili M, Zehtabchi S. Management of traumatic occult pneumothorax. Resuscitation. 2010;81(9):1063–8. Review.

Marcos Chesi de Oliveira Jr, Leonardo Yoshida Osaku,
Mariana F. Jucá Moscardi, Jonathan Parks,
and Louis Pizano

15.1 Introduction

Trauma is the main cause of death in young adults in Brazil. Increasing urban violence and the rise in the number of car accidents are to blame for increasing incidence of thoracic trauma in the young population.

Gunshot wounds to the chest can be a diagnostic challenge, as the trajectory of bullets once they enter the body is not linear, with tumbling, shattering, and reflection of the bullet. Even with an entry and exit wound, the internal injuries frequently lie outside of a straight path and relying on these can be misleading.

Similarly, in stab wounds, a small break in the skin can mask significant injury. Knives and other sharp objects vary in size and length, and the trajectory and motion of the object can lead to diagnostic confusion in the trauma bay. The clinician must maintain a high degree of suspicion for injury to distant cavities and organs during evaluation.

M. C. de Oliveira Jr
Department of Surgery, Hospital do Trabalhador Trauma Center,
Federal University of Parana, Curitiba, Brazil

L. Y. Osaku
Iwan Collaço Trauma Research Group, Department of Surgery, Hospital do Trabalhador
Trauma Center, Federal University of Parana, Curitiba, Brazil

M. F. Jucá Moscardi (✉)
University of Miami, Ryder Trauma Center, Miami, FL, USA

J. Parks
Ryder Trauma Center – Jackson Health System, Miami, FL, USA

Miller School of Medicine, University of Miami, Miami, FL, USA

L. Pizano
Division of Trauma Surgery & Critical Care, DeWitt Daughtry Family Department of
Surgery, Miller School of Medicine, University of Miami, Miami, FL, USA

© Springer Nature Switzerland AG 2020
A. Nasr et al. (eds.), *The Trauma Golden Hour*,
https://doi.org/10.1007/978-3-030-26443-7_15

This section aims to provide the clinician with an algorithmic approach to the initial evaluation of the patient with penetrating thoracic trauma in the trauma bay. In addition, it touches on the principles of observation and management of chest tubes. The operative management of penetrating thoracic injuries is beyond the scope of this text and is discussed elsewhere.

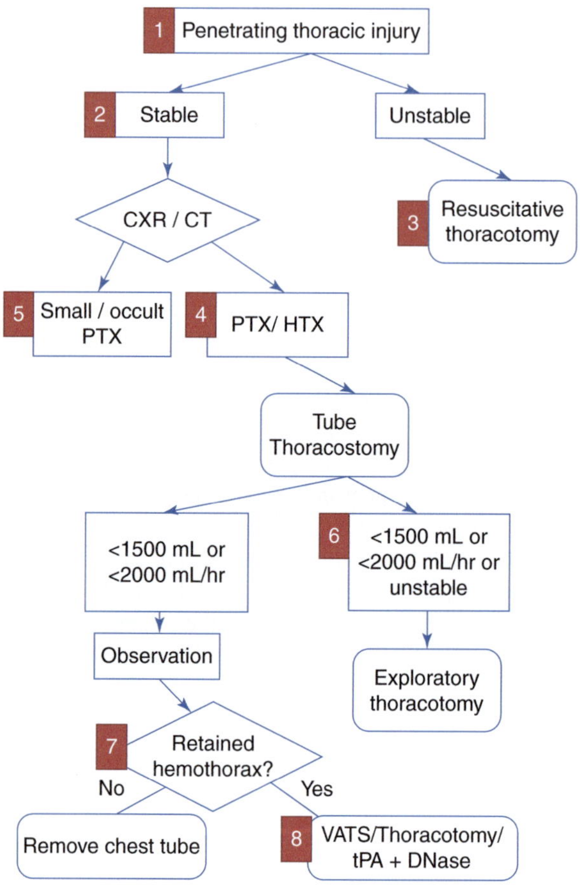

15.2 Conclusion

(1) As in other causes of trauma, evaluation of the patient with a penetrating thoracic injury begins with the primary survey of Advanced Trauma Life Support (ATLS) of the American College of Surgeons. The primary survey of the patient begins with assessment of the airway. The airway must be secured which may require intubation if necessary. Breathing is then assessed with auscultation of the lungs, and monitoring of the respiratory rate and oxygen saturation. After ensuring that the patient is ventilating and oxygenating adequately, assessment

of circulation is performed; vital signs are obtained, intravenous access is established, and any sources of hemorrhage are identified and controlled. In the case of penetrating chest trauma, this algorithmic assessment may be interrupted by the need for tube thoracostomy or thoracotomy, depending on the status of the patient.

(2) For the hemodynamically stable patient with penetrating chest trauma, the practitioner should give careful consideration for injury to the thoracic structures immediately following the primary survey. During the assessment, any change in the patient's clinical status should prompt reassessment according to the ATLS algorithm, starting again with airway, breathing, and circulation. First, a chest radiograph should be obtained to determine the presence of a hemothorax or pneumothorax. Hemothorax should be drained via tube thoracostomy promptly. Small pneumothorax can be observed in select patients with no other injuries; however, the threshold to place a chest tube for pneumothorax should be low.

After the chest radiograph and assessment for the need for a chest tube, injury to the intrathoracic structures (heart, great vessels, esophagus, trachea, bronchial tree, and lungs) is considered. This can be evaluated with computed tomography of the chest with contrast, echocardiogram, bronchoscopy, and esophagoscopy or barium swallow. A chest injury below the level of the nipple (spinal level T4) is considered a thoracoabdominal injury, and injury to the abdominal viscera and diaphragm must also be considered. Depending on the results of the completed workup, the need for specific treatment can be determined.

(3) For the hemodynamically unstable patient with penetrating chest injury, the trauma team must act quickly to determine the etiology. Consideration should be given for bleeding in the chest from a cardiac or great vessel injury, tension pneumothorax, or cardiac tamponade.

Resuscitative or "ED" thoracotomy is reserved for patients with penetrating chest trauma who are in extremis or who have loss of vital signs within 15 minutes of evaluation by the trauma team. The procedure allows for relief of tamponade, cross-clamping of the descending thoracic aorta to preserve perfusion to the heart and brain, and for direct cardiac massage. It allows for additional time for massive transfusion and transfer to the operating room for identification and definitive control and repair of the injury.

In the setting of blunt trauma, the mortality rate of patients who undergo resuscitative thoracotomy is very high, and thus the role for this procedure in blunt trauma is extremely limited, and usually performed only when the patient cardiac arrest in the presence of the provider.

(4) In the unstable patient with penetrating chest trauma, tension pneumothorax is likely and must be ruled out or relieved emergently via tube thoracostomy. In the setting where tube thoracostomy would be delayed for lack of immediate access to instruments, materials, or supplies, a needle decompression can be performed. Upon placement of the chest tube, a chest radiograph should be obtained immediately to confirm proper placement and resolution of the

pneumothorax or hemothorax. After confirmation, the primary survey begins again, with reassessment of the airway, etc.

(5) Not all pneumothoraces necessarily warrant a chest tube. Hemodynamically stable patients with penetrating chest trauma who are found to have a small pneumothorax on chest radiography or an occult pneumothorax on computed tomography may be observed as long as they do not require positive pressure ventilation, which can convert a small pneumothorax into a tension pneumothorax. These patients should be followed up closely for signs of change in breathing, oxygenation, and slight changes in vital signs before hypotension occurs, and with serial chest radiography.

(6) Upon placement of a chest tube for hemothorax, the amount of blood drained from the chest is measured and observed over time. Initial output of 1500 mL of blood or more than 200 mL per hour for 4 hours is classically used as an indicator for uncontrolled hemorrhage and a guideline for taking the patient to the operating room for an exploratory thoracotomy, though the clinical status of the patient and the clinician's judgment also play a role.

(7) Patients with chest tubes are admitted and observed for a minimum of 24–48 hours. The chest tube is evaluated daily for amount and quality of drainage, functional status, and for air leak. A daily chest X-ray should also be obtained. Once the pneumothorax is resolved or the hemothorax is drained, the chest tube can be advanced to water seal (taken off suction).

For pneumothorax, the lung, bronchial, or chest wall injury leading to the pneumothorax will take some time to heal. Healing of the leak is evidenced by lack of air leak and absence of reaccumulation of the pneumothorax after the chest tube is placed on water seal. Once the clinician is confident that the injury is healed, the chest tube may be removed. This course usually takes 48–72 hours.

For hemothorax, the quality of the drainage from the chest usually changes over time from sanguineous to serosanguineous or serous. Once this drainage is below roughly 150 mL of pleural fluid per day, and the chest X-ray demonstrates complete drainage of the pleural fluid, the chest tube may be removed.

During and immediately after removal of the chest tube, the patient is at risk of developing a pneumothorax. A chest radiograph should be obtained within an hour of removal to screen for pneumothorax, which happens approximately 10% of the time. Depending on the size of the pneumothorax and the patient's clinical status, reinsertion of the chest tube may be necessary.

(8) For undrained hemothorax or pneumothorax that will not resolve, a video-assisted thoracoscopy or thoracotomy should be considered. Patients with blood left in the pleural space are at high risk for development of empyema. An alternative that can be attempted is instillation of combination of DNAse and alteplase to break up the clot left in the chest. Several protocols for this procedure exist and vary from center to center.

Bibliography

1. Saad Junior R, de Carvalho WR, Manoel XN, Forte V. Cirurgia Torácica Geral. 2° edição. Brazil: Editora Atheneu; 2011.
2. Chiara O, Stefania C. Protocolo Para Atendimento Intra-hospitalar Do Trauma Grave. 1° Edição. Brazil: Elsevier; 2009.
3. Poggetti R, Belchor F, Birolini D. Cirurgia Do Trauma. 1° Edição. Brazil: Roca; 2006.
4. Freire E. Trauma – a Doença do Século. 1° Edição. Brazil: Editora Atheneu; 2001.
5. Marsico GA. Trauma Torácico. 1°Edição ed. Brazil: Revinter; 2006.
6. Trauma – Sociedade Panamericana De Trauma. 1° Edição. Brazil: Editora Atheneu; 2010.
7. Loogna P, Bonanno F, Bowley DM, Doll D, Girgensohn R, Smith MD, et al. Emergency thoracic surgery for penetrating, non-mediastinal trauma. ANZ J Surg. 2007;77(3):142–5.
8. Sava J, Demetriades D. Penetrating and blunt cardiac trauma: diagnosis and management. Emerg Med Australas. 2000;12(2):95–102.
9. Burack JH, Kandil E, Sawas A, O'Neill P, Sclafani SJ, Lowery RC, et al. Triage and outcome of patients with mediastinal penetrating trauma. Ann Thorac Surg. 2007;83(2):377–82; discussion 382.
10. Mollberg NM, Glenn C, John J, Wise SR, Sullivan R, Vafa A, et al. Appropriate use of emergency department thoracotomy: implications for the thoracic surgeon. Ann Thorac Surg. 2011;92(2):455–61.
11. Degiannis E, Loogna P, Doll D, Bonanno F, Bowley DM, Smith MD. Penetrating cardiac injuries: recent experience in South Africa. World J Surg. 2006;30(7):1258–64.

Main Airway Trauma

16

Ana Luisa Bettega, Glauco Afonso Morgenstern,
João Victor Pruner Vieira, Janaina de Oliveira Poy,
April Anne Grant, and Joyce Kaufman

16.1 Introduction

Main airway trauma consists in the injury of one or more segments of the anatomical region that comprises the larynx, trachea, and primary bronchi. It represents a potentially fatal severity, resulting in up to 75% mortality rate before the patient arrives at the hospital. Most of the lesions occur due to penetrating trauma, and less frequently, blunt trauma; lesions can also occur because of instrumentation of the airway, inhaling of toxic smoke or hot air, and ingestion of caustic substances. Injuries to the tracheobronchial tree are often associated with hemothorax, pneumothorax, vascular lesions, esophageal lesions, and cervical spine lesions.

Symptoms such as dyspnea, hoarseness, air leak by the penetrating wound, cervical or facial subcutaneous emphysema, and hemopneumothorax can be present in the main airway trauma. Several times, the diagnosis can be suspected by chest

A. L. Bettega (✉) · J. V. P. Vieira
Iwan Collaço Trauma Research Group, Department of Surgery, Hospital do Trabalhador
Trauma Center, Federal University of Parana, Curitiba, Brazil

G. A. Morgenstern
Department of Surgery, Hospital do Trabalhador Trauma Center,
Federal University of Parana, Curitiba, Brazil

J. de Oliveira Poy
Faculdade de Ciências Médicas de Santos, Santos, São Paulo, Brazil

A. A. Grant
Ryder Trauma Center – Jackson Health System, Miller School of Medicine, University of
Miami, Miami, FL, USA

J. Kaufman
Division of Trauma Surgery & Critical Care, DeWitt Daughtry Family Department of
Surgery, Miller School of Medicine, University of Miami, Miami, FL, USA

© Springer Nature Switzerland AG 2020
A. Nasr et al. (eds.), *The Trauma Golden Hour*,
https://doi.org/10.1007/978-3-030-26443-7_16

X-ray due to the presence of pneumomediastinum or pneumothorax. Bronchoscopy is the best method not only to localize the lesion but also to define its extension. In selected cases, it can still be necessary to perform a contrasted esophagogram, arteriography, and computed tomography, for the assessment of possible associated injuries.

Early diagnosis with immediate stabilization of the airway is the fundamental principle in the initial management of a main airway trauma, which can be done by endotracheal intubation or performing a surgical airway. The need of a surgical intervention to reconstruct the airway will be determined by the site of the injury, and also by its extension and the presence of associated lesions. Different techniques allow a satisfactory exposition of specific segments of the airway, and also an adequate reconstruction when required. Among the most common surgical complications in the treatment of main airway injuries is anastomosis dehiscence, followed by the formation of a fistula or not, late stenosis, secondary to the healing process of the injury. When these complications occur, a new fibrobronchoscopy and, if necessary, another surgical procedure is recommended.

Tracheobronchial lesions are uncommon and have high lethality; it is possible to get good results with the early treatment of the patients who survive until they arrive at an emergency service.

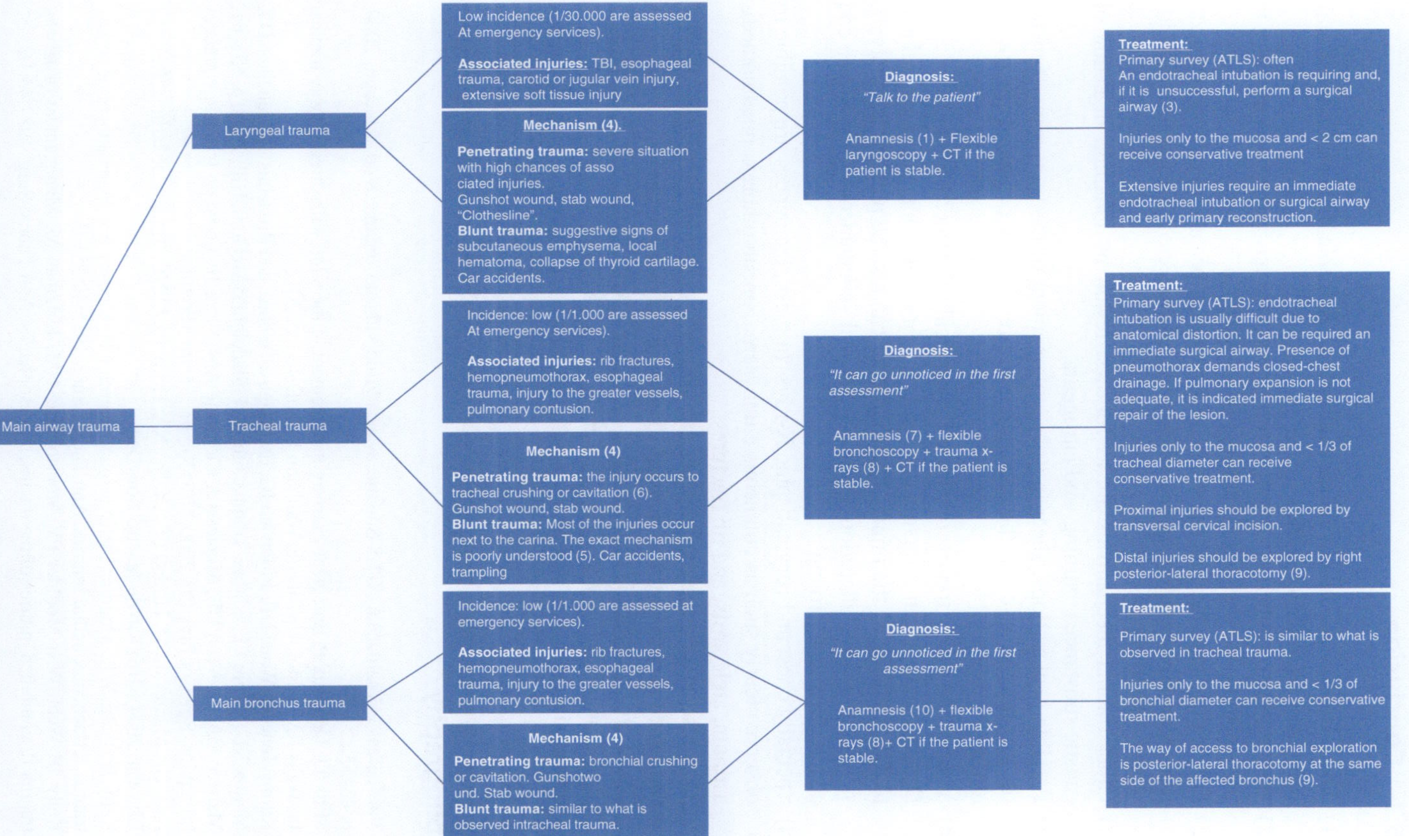

Main airway trauma

Laryngeal trauma

Low incidence (1/30.000 are assessed
At emergency services).
Associated injuries: TBI, esophageal
trauma, carotid or jugular vein injury,
extensive soft tissue injury

Mechanism (4).
Penetrating trauma: severe situation
with high chances of asso
ciated injuries.
Gunshot wound, stab wound,
"Clothesline".
Blunt trauma: suggestive signs of
subcutaneous emphysema, local
hematoma, collapse of thyroid cartilage.
Car accidents.

Diagnosis:
"Talk to the patient"
Anamnesis (1) + Flexible
laryngoscopy + CT if the
patient is stable.

Treatment:
Primary survey (ATLS): often
An endotracheal intubation is requiring and,
if it is unsuccessful, perform a surgical
airway (3).
Injuries only to the mucosa and < 2 cm can
receive conservative treatment
Extensive injuries require an immediate
endotracheal intubation or surgical airway
and early primary reconstruction.

Tracheal trauma

Incidence: low (1/1.000 are assessed
At emergency services).
Associated injuries: rib fractures,
hemopneumothorax, esophageal
trauma, injury to the greater vessels,
pulmonary contusion.

Mechanism (4)
Penetrating trauma: the injury occurs to
tracheal crushing or cavitation (6).
Gunshot wound, stab wound.
Blunt trauma: Most of the injuries occur
next to the carina. The exact mechanism
is poorly understood (5). Car accidents,
trampling

Diagnosis:
"It can go unnoticed in the first
assessment"
Anamnesis (7) + flexible
bronchoscopy + trauma x-
rays (8) + CT if the patient is
stable.

Treatment:
Primary survey (ATLS): endotracheal
intubation is usually difficult due to
anatomical distortion. It can be required an
immediate surgical airway. Presence of
pneumothorax demands closed-chest
drainage. If pulmonary expansion is not
adequate, it is indicated immediate surgical
repair of the lesion.
Injuries only to the mucosa and < 1/3 of
tracheal diameter can receive
conservative treatment.
Proximal injuries should be explored by
transversal cervical incision.
Distal injuries should be explored by right
posterior-lateral thoracotomy (9).

Main bronchus trauma

Incidence: low (1/1.000 are assessed at
emergency services).
Associated injuries: rib fractures,
hemopneumothorax, esophageal
trauma, injury to the greater vessels,
pulmonary contusion.

Mechanism (4)
Penetrating trauma: bronchial crushing
or cavitation. Gunshotwo
und. Stab wound.
Blunt trauma: similar to what is
observed intracheal trauma.

Diagnosis:
"It can go unnoticed in the first
assessment"
Anamnesis (10) + flexible
bronchoscopy + trauma x-
rays (8)+ CT if the patient is
stable.

Treatment:
Primary survey (ATLS): is similar to what is
observed in tracheal trauma.
Injuries only to the mucosa and < 1/3 of
bronchial diameter can receive conservative
treatment.
The way of access to bronchial exploration
is posterior-lateral thoracotomy at the same
side of the affected bronchus (9).

16.2   Conclusion

(1) Triad: Hoarseness, subcutaneous emphysema, palpable fracture. Dyspnea may be present in different grades.

(2) Endotracheal intubation: it can be orotracheal or nasotracheal, according to the situation and the level of training of the surgeon.

(3) Surgical airway: the first option is tracheostomy, because it allows stabilization of the airway below the site of the injury. In selected cases, a cricothyroidotomy can be performed.

(4) Other trauma mechanisms are as follows: lesion by inhaling, ingestion of caustic substances, burning, and iatrogenia.

(5) Possible explanations: shear injuries, enlargement of the transverse diameter of the thorax, rise of the intrathoracic pressure associated with glottal closure.

(6) Most of the times, trauma occurs in the cervical trachea (75–80%).

(7) Dyspnea is the main symptom in most of the cases; it is not necessarily related to the extension of the injury. The following can also be present: hemoptysis, stridor, and voice alteration. Facial or cervical subcutaneous emphysema can also be frequently found.

(8) Specially chest and cervical spine X-rays. In these, incidences are possible to observe clearly such as cutaneous emphysema, pneumothorax, pneumomediastinum, atelectasis, and rib fractures.

(9) The presence of associated injuries can affect the choice of the surgeon regarding which access way will be used to explore the thoracic cavity.

(10) The main symptom is also dyspnea associated with hemoptysis, stridor, and alteration of the voice. The presence of an associated pneumothorax is common.

Bibliography

1. Vias aéreas e Ventilação. ATLS-Suporte avançado de vida no trauma. 8ªed. Chicago; 2008. p. 43–53.
2. Mills TJ, Deblieux P. Emergency airway management in the adult with direct airway trauma. In: Walls RM, editor. UpToDate. Waltham: UpToDate Inc; 2012
3. Karmy-Jones R, Wood DE, Jurkovich JG. Esophagus, Trachea, and Bronchus. In: Feliciano DV, Mattox KL, Moore EE, editors. Trauma. 6th ed. Philadelphia: McGraw-Hill; 2008. p. 553–61.
4. Marsico GA, Azevedo DE, Montessi J, Clemente AM, Viera JP. Lesão da traqueia e grandes bronquios. Rev Col Bras Cir. 2000;27(3) Rio de Janeiro May/June.
5. Faga GP, Mantovani M, Hirano ES, Crespo NA, Horovitz APNC. Trauma de laringe. Rev Col Bras Cir. 2004;31(6) Rio de Janeiro Nov./Dec.
6. Kelly JP, Webb WR, Moulder PV, Everson C, Burch BH, Lindsey ES. Management of airway trauma I: tracheobronchial injuries. Ann Thorac Surg. 1985;40:551–5.
7. Kelly JP, Webb WR, Moulder PV, Moustouakas NM, Lirtzman M. Management of airway trauma II: combined injuries of the trachea and esophagus. Ann Thorac Surg. 1987;43:160–3.

Pulmonary Trauma

17

Marianne Reitz, Vinicius Basso Preti, Beatriz Ortis Yazbek, Ana Luisa Bettega, and Antonio Marttos

Thoracic injuries are responsible for around 20–25% of deaths by trauma, and it is an associated factor to it in other 25%. Almost one-third of affected patients present some level of thoracic injury.

17.1 Clinical Evaluation

Time is an important factor in the assessment and approach of the patient; therefore, anamnesis and physical exam should be performed fast and objectively, prioritizing the most severe injuries. Physical exam should cover inspection, palpation, percussion, and auscultation; and also be complemented by imaging exams when necessary.

Primary survey should aim the diagnosis and treatment of injuries capable of altering or disrupting ventilator exchange. These alterations should not be immediately related to parenchymal trauma, once this injury appears late. The most probable causes should be considered, such as airway obstruction, pneumothorax, secretion aspiration, and sucking chest wound.

M. Reitz · A. L. Bettega (✉)
Iwan Collaço Trauma Research Group, Department of Surgery, Hospital do Trabalhador Trauma Center, Federal University of Parana, Curitiba, Brazil

V. B. Preti
Department of Surgery, Hospital do Trabalhador Trauma Center, Federal University of Parana, Curitiba, Brazil

B. O. Yazbek
Faculdade de Ciências Médicas de Santos, Santos, São Paulo, Brazil

A. Marttos
William Lehman Injury Research Center, Division of Trauma & Surgical Critical Care, Dewitt Daughtry Department of Surgery, Leonard M. Miller School of Medicine Miami, University of Miami, Miami, FL, USA

© Springer Nature Switzerland AG 2020
A. Nasr et al. (eds.), *The Trauma Golden Hour*,
https://doi.org/10.1007/978-3-030-26443-7_17

Initially, imaging exams should be directed, with a clear and functional purpose, based on the findings of the physical exam and aiming the treatment of the suspected injuries.

Chest X-ray is the most used exam for the diagnosis of pulmonary injuries in traumatized patients, it is a fast exam that exposes the patients to a minimal amount of radiation, and it can be also used in pregnant women when necessary.

Computed tomography has earned more space and has been more used in trauma due to more modern equipment that allow faster exams. It is a better exam to confirm and quantify the lesions, and evaluate the pleural space and adjacent structures, such as base vessels, associated vascular tissue, and bone components.

17.2 Thoracic Lesions

Most common conditions related to thoracic trauma are pain, bleeding, mechanical instability of the chest wall, and defects of the chest wall.

17.3 Pain

Pain should be managed with careful and effective administration of analgesics. Although analgesics do not cause any direct effect on the stability of the wall or any functional alteration, their use can result in posterior ventilator imbalance by conscious decrease of thoracic mobility.

17.4 Pneumothorax

It is found in more than 20% of trauma in general and it is defined as an air collection in pleural space. It can be classified as simple, open, and hypertensive. Classical findings to all kinds of pneumothorax are respiratory discomfort, decrease of vesicular murmur on the affected side and hyperresonance on percussion. In hypertensive pneumothorax, there is also tracheal deviation to the opposite side of the injury, tachycardia, and jugular distention.

The size of the pneumothorax is not always related to the patient's clinical presentation, which should be prioritized in the evaluation of the treatment. A closed-chest drainage can be performed in patients with a simple pneumothorax (20–22 French tube) in the fifth or sixth intercostal space in the anterior or midaxillary line. It is preferable to place the tube in the anterior axillary line due to more posterior comfort for the patient.

A simple pneumothorax can evolve to a hypertensive pneumothorax; therefore, the patient should be always carefully monitored. As the first management procedure of a hypertensive pneumothorax, a puncture with a gauge needle (10 to 16 gauge), sufficiently long to penetrate through the chest wall in the second or third intercostal space of the affected hemithorax, in the hemiclavicular line, to an immediate decompression, should be performed, transforming the hypertensive pneumothorax into an open pneumothorax. The next step is to perform a pleural drainage. Besides, patients should receive supplementary oxygen by a mask or undergo an orotracheal intubation with mechanical ventilation when necessary. A chest X-ray should be performed after the placement of the tube to verify if it is in place and if the drainage is effective.

During pre-hospital care, sucking chest wounds should be managed with a dressing that seals the wound in three sides to create a valve mechanism (allowing the exit of the air during expiration and preventing its entrance during inspiration). During hospitalar care, the chest drainage is preconized through a different site from the wound – which should be closed by occlusive dressing or synthesis of the skin by separated stitches – and orotracheal intubation when necessary. Bigger defects should be managed surgically by thoracotomy with correction of the lesion, closed-chest drainage, and mechanical ventilation with positive pressure.

17.5 Hemothorax

The second most frequent pulmonary lesion is the hemothorax. The aim of the treatment is allowing pulmonary reexpansion, which for itself contributes to the decrease of the bleeding by compressing the pleura. Less than 10% of the cases should be treated by thoracotomy to identify and control the source of the bleeding. The rest of the cases should be treated by closed-chest drainage with tubes bigger than the ones used to treat pneumothorax (36–38 French) due to the bigger chance of occlusion by cloths and secretions. If the drainage is not sufficient, a second tube can be placed. When the chest X-ray leaves doubts and other causes of pulmonary opacification must be discarded (pulmonary contusion, hematoma, pulmonary infiltrates, pulmonary collapse by selective intubation), computed tomography should be performed. Coagulated hemothorax (which makes the drainage harder), unstable patients, and persistent bleedings should be managed surgically by thoracotomy.

17.6 Pulmonary Contusion

This is the third most common pulmonary lesion and the fourth when considering all thoracic traumas. The treatment consists in effective analgesia and adequate ventilatory support.

Pulmonary contusion may not be recognized or be underestimated during the first assessment, worsening in the first 24 hours after the trauma, resulting in around 43% of mortality.

Although it rarely requires intervention and is usually treated conservatively, treatment options to unstable patients are computed angiotomography and embolization.

17.6.1 Rib Fractures

Although this is not a specific pulmonary lesion, rib fractures can cause pulmonary laceration, altering the ventilator function. Rib fracture is the most common thoracic injury in blunt thoracic trauma, and there is a direct correlation between the number of fractured ribs, the number of associated injuries, and the morbidity. Up until 70% of the cases are related to another thoracic injury, especially hemothorax, pneumothorax, and pulmonary contusion.

17.7 Associated Injuries

Fracture or dissociation of the shoulder blade should be evaluated also by the orthopedist and vascular surgeon, because it is usually associated with nerve damage and vascular injury. The most common injuries are injury to the brachial plexus (between 13% and 81% of the cases) and of the axillar and subclavian artery (around 81% of the cases). Sternum fractures are associated with significative lesions inside and outside the thorax in 50–60% of the cases, with the most common ones being the rib fractures, long bones fractures, and skull fractures. Patients with sternum fractures by blunt trauma should be evaluated regarding the possibility of a cardiac injury.

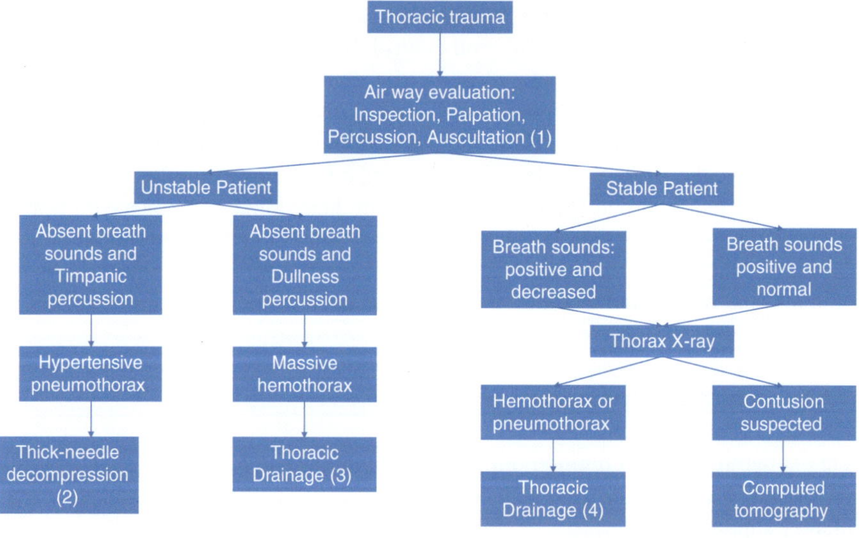

17.8 Conclusion

(1) Inspection, palpation, percussion, auscultation
(2) 10–16 gauge
(3) 36–38 French
(4) 20–22 French if pneumothorax, and 36–38 French if hemothorax

Bibliography

1. Feliciano DV, Mattox KL, Moore EE. Trauma. 6th ed: New York, NY: McGraw-Hill; 2008. p. 526–52.
2. Freire E. Trauma: a doença dos séculos. Ed Atheneu, 2001. p. 1389–94.
3. Al-Koudmani I, Darwish B, Al-Kateb K, Taifour Y. Chest trauma experience over eleven-year period at Al-Mouassat University Teaching Hospital – Damascus: a retrospective review of 888 cases. J Cardiothorac Surg. 2012;7(1):35.
4. Reaghavendran K, Notter RH, Davidson BA, Helinski JD, Kunkel SL, Knight PR. Lung contusion: inflammatory mechanisms and interaction with other injuries. Shock. 2009;32(2):122–30.
5. Aukema TS, Beenen LFM, Hietbrink F, Leenen LPH. Initial assessment of chest x-ray in thoracic trauma patients: awareness of specific injuries. Word J Radiol. 2012;4(2):48–52.
6. D'Ippolito G, Medeiros RB. Exames radiológicos na gestação. Radiol Bras. 2005;38(6):447–50.

Great Vessels and Cardiac Trauma

Marcelo Tsuyoshi Yamane, Phillipe Abreu,
Ana Luisa Bettega, Andrea Rachel Marcadis,
and Antonio Marttos

18.1 Introduction

The management of cardiac trauma depends on its etiology. While penetrating trauma most commonly causes ventricular injury, blunt cardiac trauma may result in a variety of pathologies including myocardial contusion, coronary artery injury, atrial rupture, or ventricular or valve rupture. Great vessels can also be affected by both blunt and penetrating trauma, and can result in a range of signs and symptoms, from spontaneous resolving arrhythmias to lethal transections.

The initial management of a patient with cardiac or great vessel trauma is to ensure airway and ventilation with adequate oxygenation, and treat shock according to ATLS protocol. The physician should inspect the chest for bruises, lacerations, and penetrating wounds; palpate the sternum and costal arches; and auscultate for muffled heart tones. Furthermore, it is essential to inspect the jugular veins, as these are an important part of Beck triad (muffled heart tones, hypotension, and distended jugular veins), which can be seen with cardiac tamponade. The evaluation of the peripheral pulses is also fundamental to the evaluation of a patient with suspected

M. T. Yamane · P. Abreu (⊠) · A. L. Bettega
Iwan Collaço Trauma Research Group, Department of Surgery, Hospital do Trabalhador
Trauma Center, Federal University of Parana, Curitiba, Brazil

A. R. Marcadis
Department of Surgery, University of Miami, Miller School of Medicine, Jackson Memorial
Hospital, Miami, FL, USA

A. Marttos
William Lehman Injury Research Center, Division of Trauma & Surgical Critical Care,
Dewitt Daughtry Department of Surgery, Leonard M. Miller School of Medicine Miami,
University of Miami, Miami, FL, USA

© Springer Nature Switzerland AG 2020
A. Nasr et al. (eds.), *The Trauma Golden Hour*,
https://doi.org/10.1007/978-3-030-26443-7_18

cardiac or great vessel injury. FAST is a very useful adjunct tool in cardiac trauma because it allows diagnosis of injuries in the emergency room and, when performed by an experienced user, has a sensitivity of almost 100% and a specificity of 97.3% for cardiac injury.

Penetrating Cardiac Trauma Penetrating wounds to the anatomic area known as the "cardiac box" (bordered superiorly by the clavicles, inferiorly by the xiphoid, and by the nipples laterally) should increase the suspicion of cardiac injury. Knife wounds to the cardiac box, for example, are associated with an up to 80% risk of cardiac tamponade. The Beck triad, paradoxical pulses, and Kussmaul sign (paradoxical rise or failure of the appropriate fall in jugular venous pressure on inspiration) are seen in a minority of patients with cardiac tamponade; hence, it is important not to depend on these signs if the diagnosis is suspected. Firearm injuries to the heart are more often associated with bleeding and exsanguination rather than tamponade. Definitive treatment involves surgical exposure through an anterior thoracotomy or median sternotomy with subsequent tamponade relief and/or hemorrhage control. After the chest is exposed, the pericardium anterior to the phrenic nerve is opened, injuries are identified, and repair is performed. During cardiorrhaphy, a Foley catheter or a skin stapler can be used to tamponade the injury as a temporary measure for hemostasis. Removal of bullets should be performed only when they are in the left chambers, larger than 1–2 cm, irregularly shaped, or produce symptoms.

Blunt Heart Trauma The primary management of blunt cardiac injury (BCI) is supportive care. In patients requiring blood pressure or cardiac output support, inotropes can be very effective. Transvenous cardiac pacing may also be a useful tool when there is a high-grade atrioventricular block after myocardial contusion. Surgical intervention for BCI is rarely required. The role of surgery in BCI should be restricted to patients with structural abnormalities and/or a positive FAST; in these patients, a pericardial window should be rapidly performed. The patient should be prepared for the possibility of extending the incision to a median sternotomy if there is hemopericardium. Extracorporeal circulation and/or valve replacements may be necessary in the treatment of complex intracardiac lesions.

Trauma of Great Vessels Injury to large vessels such as the aorta, brachiocephalic branches, pulmonary arteries and veins, vena cava, innominate veins, and azygos vein can occur with both blunt and penetrating trauma. More than 90% of the lesions of the great thoracic vessels occur due to penetrating trauma, while the vessels most susceptible to blunt trauma are the descending thoracic aorta, innominate artery, pulmonary veins, and vena cava. The clinical picture of great vessel trauma includes hypotension, unequal arterial pressures or pulses in the extremities, external evidence of major thoracic trauma, and palpable fracture of the sternum or thoracic spine. Exsanguination from these injuries can occur either acutely, or in the chronic phase in the presence of a fistula involving an adjacent structure or rupture of a post-traumatic pseudoaneurysm.

Indications for emergency thoracotomy include hemodynamic instability, significant bleeding in the thoracic drains, or radiographic evidence of a rapidly expanding mediastinal hematoma. Selecting the incision is critical to gaining adequate exposure. For the hypotensive patient with an undiagnosed lesion, left antero-lateral thoracotomy should be performed. In stable patients, findings on preoperative arteriography may dictate an operative approach by another incision. Conventional open repair of traumatic aortic rupture with interposition graft is the standard technique, as it is safe, effective, and durable. Simple aortic cross-clamping, the "clamp and sew" technique, has been used in the past, but is associated with higher rates of paraplegia than techniques that use extracorporeal lower body perfusion.

Thoracic endovascular aortic repair (TEVAR) is more commonly used for patients with significant comorbidities; however, in some hospitals, TEVAR has become the preferred treatment for blunt aortic injury. Endovascular repair is associated with a significant decrease in mortality and lower incidence of spinal cord ischemia compared to open surgical repair.

Subclavian vessel lesions may be controlled by packing or intravascular balloon catheters. Hemorrhage from the pulmonary wire can be controlled by proximal clamping of the wire or by twisting the lung 180°. In thoracic vena cava injuries, repair should be performed through the right atrium.

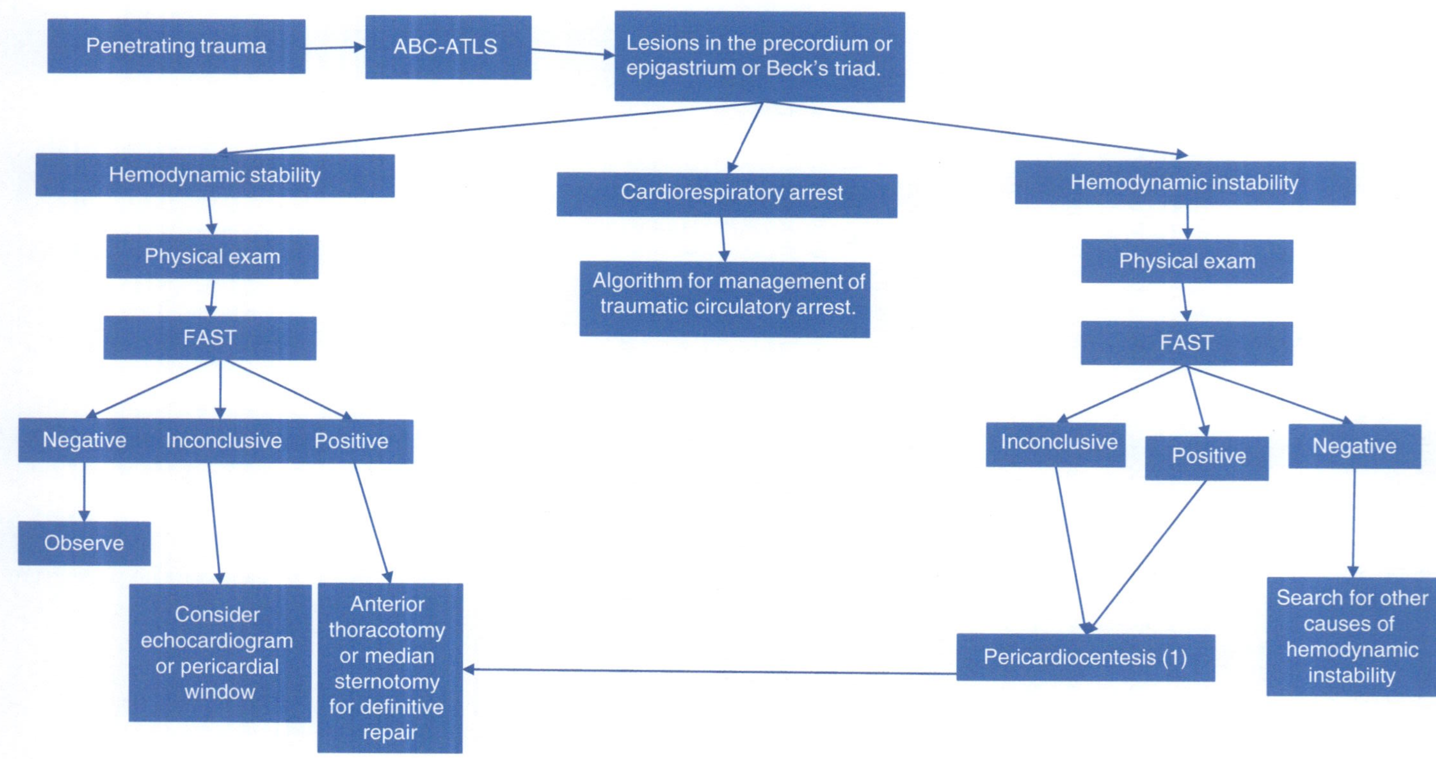

Penetrating trauma
ABC-ATLS
Lesions in the precordium or epigastrium or Beck's triad.
Hemodynamic stability
Cardiorespiratory arrest
Hemodynamic instability
Physical exam
Algorithm for management of traumatic circulatory arrest.
Physical exam
FAST
FAST
Negative
Inconclusive
Positive
Inconclusive
Positive
Negative
Observe
Consider echocardiogram or pericardial window
Anterior thoracotomy or median sternotomy for definitive repair
Pericardiocentesis (1)
Search for other causes of hemodynamic instability

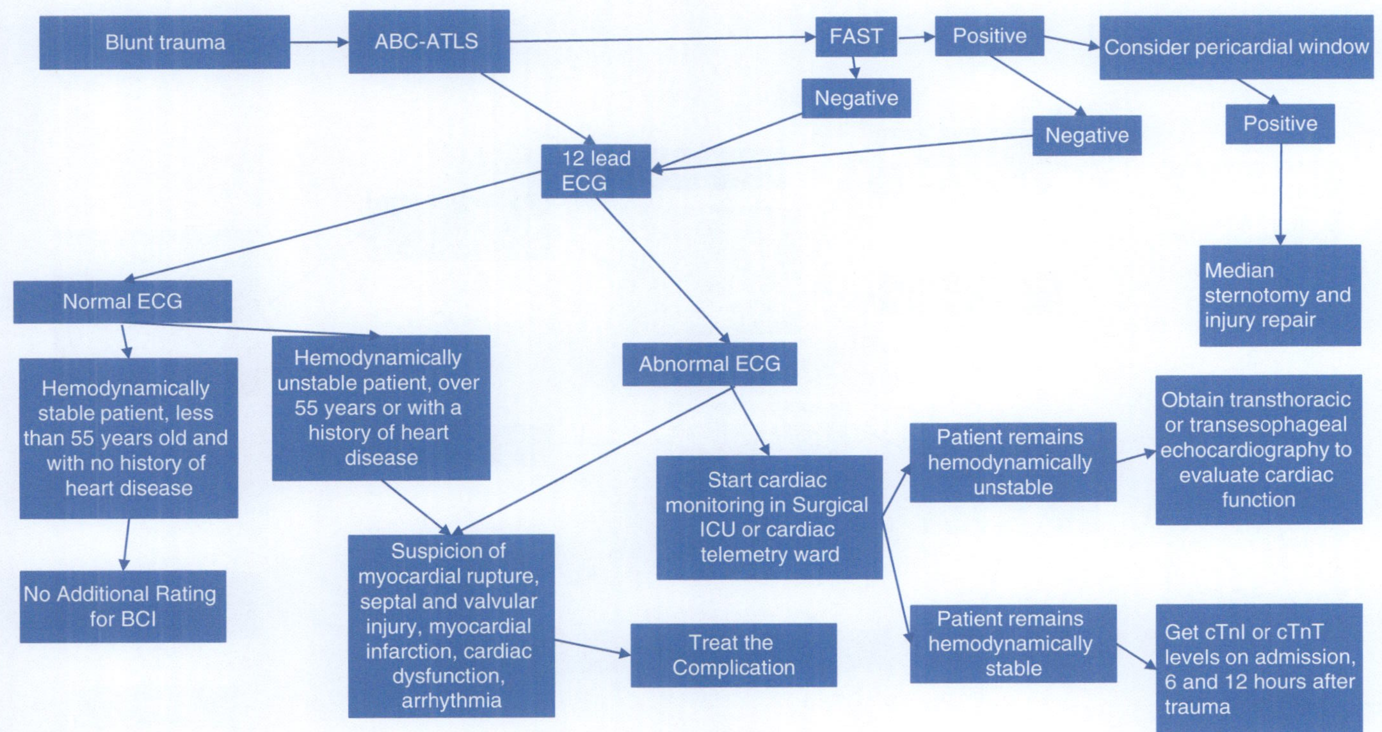

Blunt trauma
ABC-ATLS
FAST
Positive
Negative
Consider pericardial window
Positive
Negative
Median sternotomy and injury repair
12 lead ECG
Normal ECG
Abnormal ECG
Hemodynamically stable patient, less than 55 years old and with no history of heart disease
Hemodynamically unstable patient, over 55 years or with a history of heart disease
No Additional Rating for BCI
Suspicion of myocardial rupture, septal and valvular injury, myocardial infarction, cardiac dysfunction, arrhythmia
Start cardiac monitoring in Surgical ICU or cardiac telemetry ward
Treat the Complication
Patient remains hemodynamically unstable
Patient remains hemodynamically stable
Obtain transthoracic or transesophageal echocardiography to evaluate cardiac function
Get cTnI or cTnT levels on admission, 6 and 12 hours after trauma

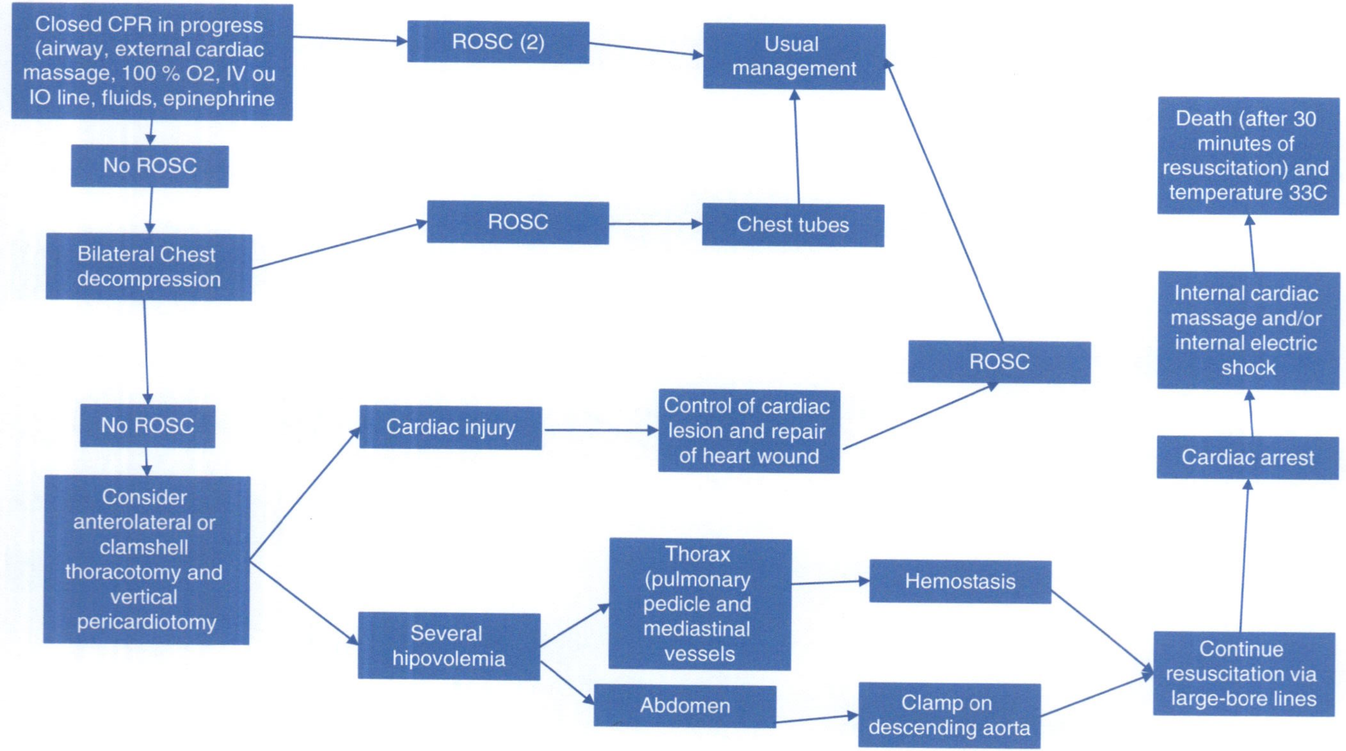
Closed CPR in progress (airway, external cardiac massage, 100 % O2, IV ou IO line, fluids, epinephrine
ROSC (2)
Usual management
No ROSC
Bilateral Chest decompression
ROSC
Chest tubes
No ROSC
Cardiac injury
Control of cardiac lesion and repair of heart wound
ROSC
Consider anterolateral or clamshell thoracotomy and vertical pericardiotomy
Several hipovolemia
Thorax (pulmonary pedicle and mediastinal vessels
Hemostasis
Abdomen
Clamp on descending aorta
Continue resuscitation via large-bore lines
Cardiac arrest
Internal cardiac massage and/or internal electric shock
Death (after 30 minutes of resuscitation) and temperature 33C

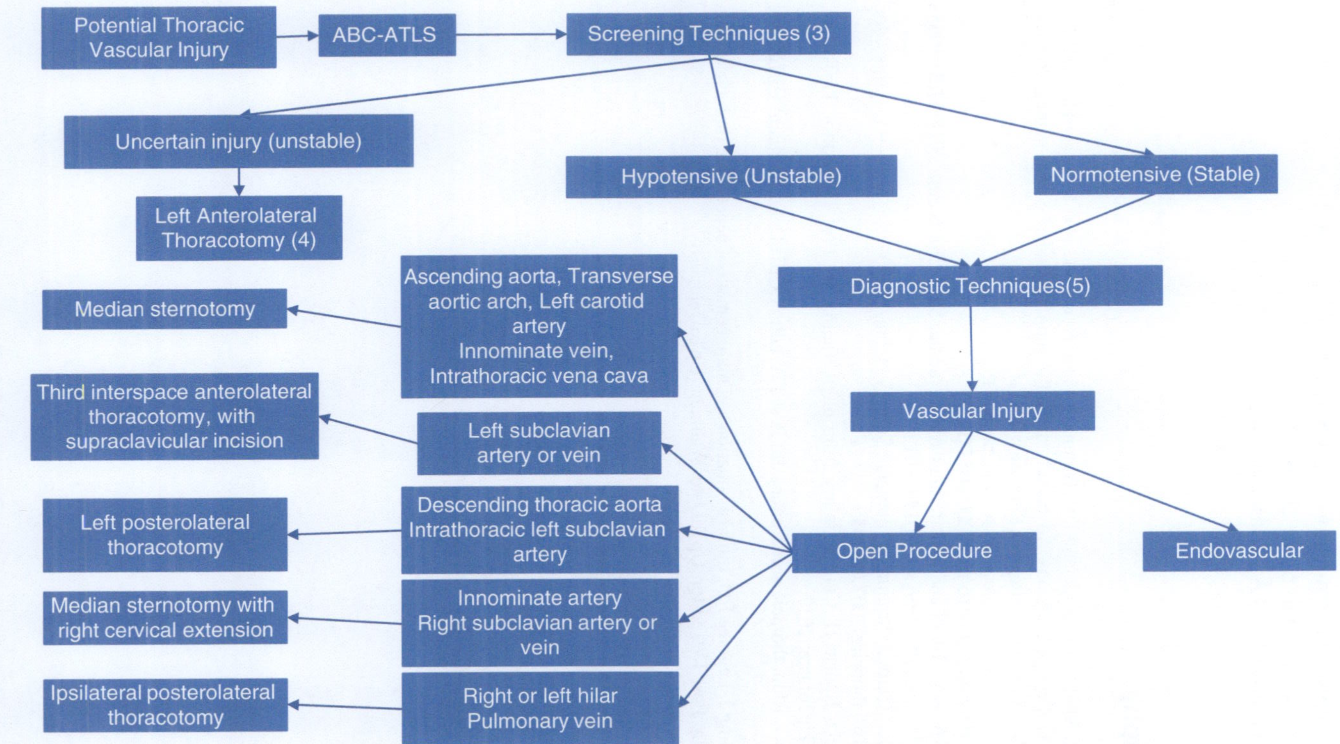

Potential Thoracic Vascular Injury
ABC-ATLS
Screening Techniques (3)
Uncertain injury (unstable)
Hypotensive (Unstable)
Normotensive (Stable)
Left Anterolateral Thoracotomy (4)
Diagnostic Techniques(5)
Ascending aorta, Transverse aortic arch, Left carotid artery Innominate vein, Intrathoracic vena cava
Median sternotomy
Vascular Injury
Third interspace anterolateral thoracotomy, with supraclavicular incision
Left subclavian artery or vein
Left posterolateral thoracotomy
Descending thoracic aorta Intrathoracic left subclavian artery
Open Procedure
Endovascular
Median sternotomy with right cervical extension
Innominate artery Right subclavian artery or vein
Ipsilateral posterolateral thoracotomy
Right or left hilar Pulmonary vein

(1) Do when it is not possible to perform thoracotomy.
(2) ROSC = Return of spontaneous circulation.
(3) History, physical examination, chest X-ray, FAST, chest CT.
(4) Consider extension to right "clamshell."
(5) Tube thoracostomy, FAST, arteriogram.

Bibliography

1. Moore EE, Mattox KL, Feliciano DV. Trauma. 8nd ed. New York, NY: McGraw-Hill; 2017.
2. American College of Surgeons. Advanced trauma life support: student course manual. 10th ed. Chicago, IL: American College of Surgeons; 2017.
3. Cook CC, Gleason TG. Great vessel and cardiac trauma. Surg Clin N Am. 2009;89(4):797–820. https://doi.org/10.1016/j.suc.2009.05.002.
4. Bellister SA, et al. Blunt and penetrating cardiac trauma. Surg Clin N Am. 2017;97(5):1065–76. https://doi.org/10.1016/j.suc.2017.06.012.
5. Embrey R. Cardiac trauma. Thoracic Surgery Clinics. 2007;17(1):87–93. https://doi.org/10.1016/j.thorsurg.2007.02.002.
6. Legome ED, Kadish H. Cardiac injury from blunt trauma. In: Post TW, editor. UpToDate. Waltham: UpToDate; 2017.
7. Neschis DG. Blunt thoracic aortic injury. In: Post TW, editor. UpToDate. Waltham: UpToDate; 2017.
8. Mayglothling J, Legome ED. Initial evaluation and management of penetrating thoracic trauma in adults. In: Post TW, editor. UpToDate. Waltham: UpToDate; 2017.

Esophageal Trauma

19

Ana Gabriela Clemente, João Henrique Felicio de Lima,
Beatriz Ortis Yazbek, Ana Luisa Bettega,
and Antonio Marttos

Esophageal injuries are a challenge to surgeons due to their complex presentation, diagnosis, and treatment. In spite of improved surgical techniques, new diagnostic modalities, and therapeutic advancements, morbidity and mortality rates remain high. Isolated esophageal trauma is rare and is usually related to other organic lesions. Complications include stenosis, fistula (10–28%), wound infection, mediastinitis, empyema, pneumonia, and sepsis.

A. G. Clemente · A. L. Bettega (✉)
Iwan Collaço Trauma Research Group, Department of Surgery, Hospital do Trabalhador
Trauma Center, Federal University of Parana, Curitiba, Brazil

J. H. F. de Lima
Department of Surgery, Hospital do Trabalhador Trauma Center,
Federal University of Parana, Curitiba, Brazil

B. O. Yazbek
Faculdade de Ciências Médicas de Santos, Santos, São Paulo, Brazil

A. Marttos
William Lehman Injury Research Center, Division of Trauma & Surgical Critical Care,
Dewitt Daughtry Department of Surgery, Leonard M. Miller School of Medicine Miami,
University of Miami, Miami, FL, USA

© Springer Nature Switzerland AG 2020

A. Nasr et al. (eds.), *The Trauma Golden Hour*,
https://doi.org/10.1007/978-3-030-26443-7_19

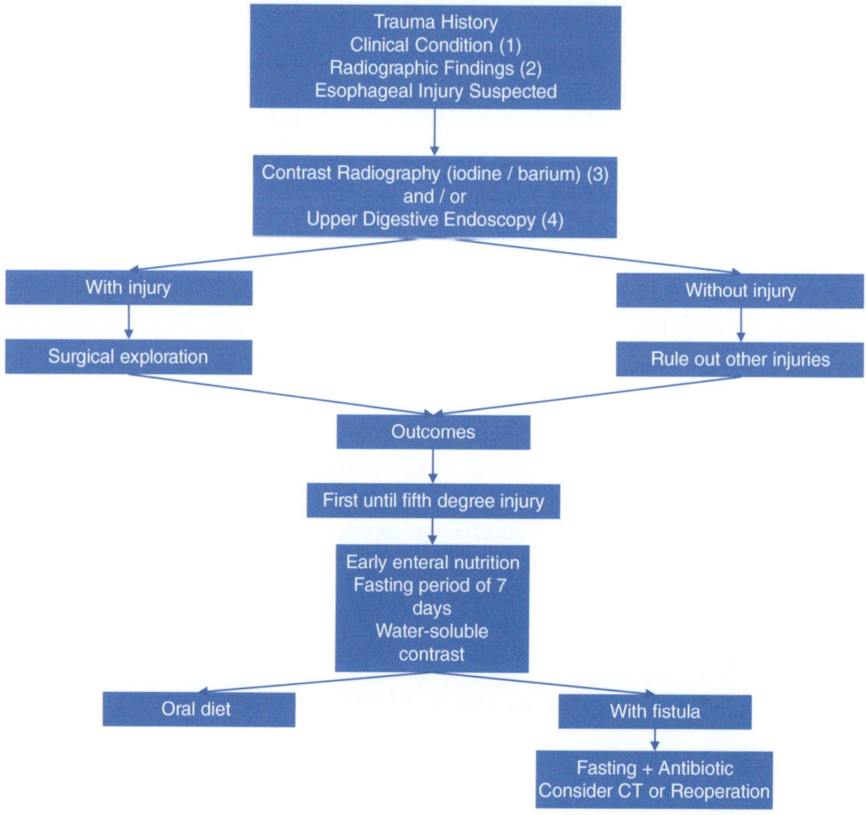
Trauma History
Clinical Condition (1)
Radiographic Findings (2)
Esophageal Injury Suspected

Contrast Radiography (iodine / barium) (3)
and / or
Upper Digestive Endoscopy (4)

With injury

Without injury

Surgical exploration

Rule out other injuries

Outcomes

First until fifth degree injury

Early enteral nutrition
Fasting period of 7
days
Water-soluble
contrast

Oral diet

With fistula

Fasting + Antibiotic
Consider CT or Reoperation

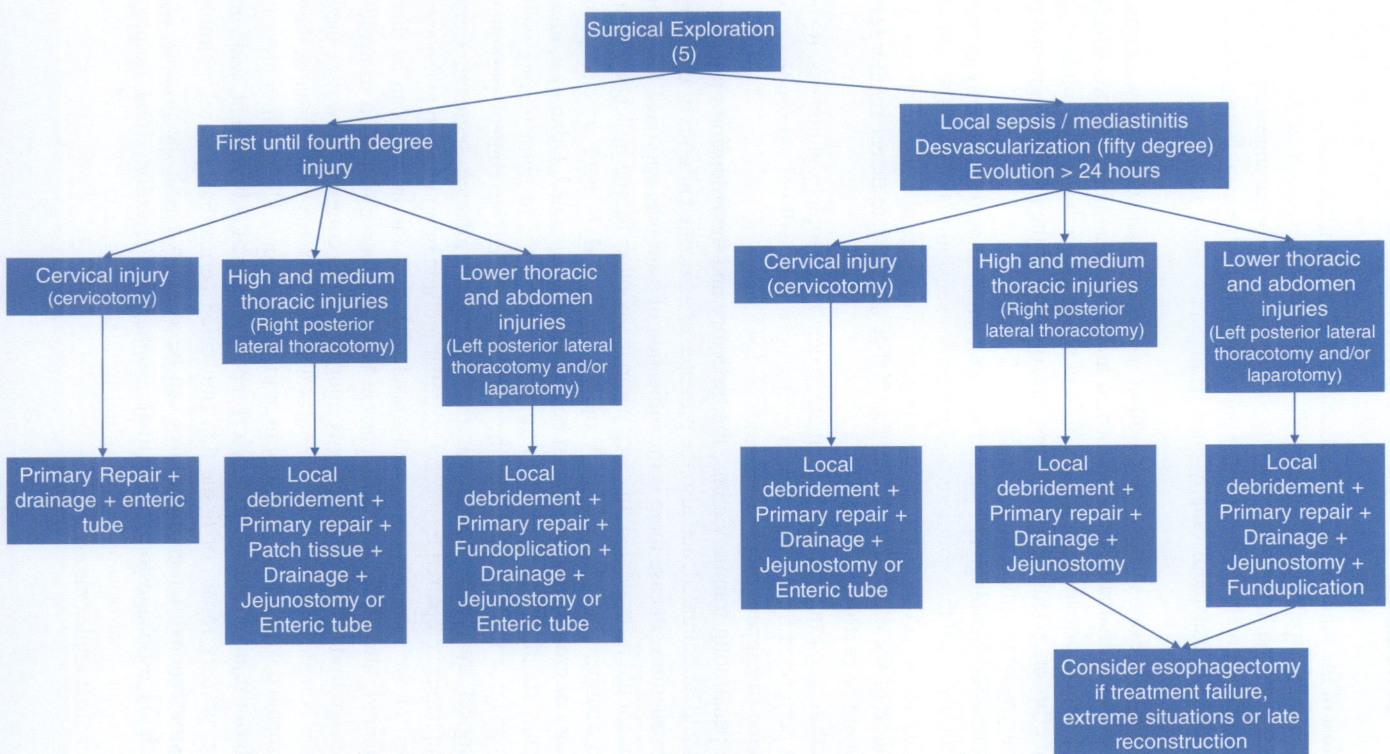

Surgical Exploration (5)
First until fourth degree injury
Local sepsis / mediastinitis Desvascularization (fifty degree) Evolution > 24 hours
Cervical injury (cervicotomy)
High and medium thoracic injuries (Right posterior lateral thoracotomy)
Lower thoracic and abdomen injuries (Left posterior lateral thoracotomy and/or laparotomy)
Cervical injury (cervicotomy)
High and medium thoracic injuries (Right posterior lateral thoracotomy)
Lower thoracic and abdomen injuries (Left posterior lateral thoracotomy and/or laparotomy)
Primary Repair + drainage + enteric tube
Local debridement + Primary repair + Patch tissue + Drainage + Jejunostomy or Enteric tube
Local debridement + Primary repair + Fundoplication + Drainage + Jejunostomy or Enteric tube
Local debridement + Primary repair + Drainage + Jejunostomy or Enteric tube
Local debridement + Primary repair + Drainage + Jejunostomy
Local debridement + Primary repair + Drainage + Jejunostomy + Funduplication
Consider esophagectomy if treatment failure, extreme situations or late reconstruction

19.1 Conclusion

(1) Most of the injuries are due to penetrating trauma and are in the cervical region. Clinical symptoms are found in 60–80% of the cases; the most frequent symptoms are dysphagia, odynophagia, hematemesis, oropharyngeal bleeding, subcutaneous emphysema, cervical pain, chest pain, dyspnea, hoarseness, cough, stridor, mediastinum emphysema (Hamman's sign), and saliva or secretion output.

(2) Diagnostic evaluation is composed of radiological and endoscopic exams. The first exams that should be performed are cervical and chest X-ray, which can present abnormalities in around 80% of the cases, such as pneumothorax, pleural effusion, pneumomediastinum, enlargement of the mediastinum, and retropharyngeal of subcutaneous tissue air dissection.

(3) Contrasted radiological exam of the esophagus should be initially performed with water-soluble solutions and presents a sensibility of 62–100% and specificity of 94–100%. After having a negative radiological exam, a barium examination of the esophagus, which has higher accuracy to detect smaller lesions, should be performed.

(4) Endoscopic exam is used to evaluate in detail the esophageal mucosa. It should be performed by an experienced endoscopist who will not worsen the existing lesion (it happens in 1% of cases).

(5) In penetrating trauma victims, the trajectory and the extension on the wound should be evaluated, and also the presence of associated injuries of other organs or structures. In case there is the indication of a surgical approach, the esophagus should be evaluated. In cases without any other formal indication of surgical treatment, esophageal injury must be discarded. If there are clear signs of injury or great suspicion, it must be immediately operated. Otherwise, imaging exams should be performed to guide the diagnosis. In blunt trauma victims, esophageal evaluation should be performed based on clinical presentation. Surgical treatment depends on the esophageal affected segment. Cervical esophagus is repaired by a cervical collar incision or an incision at the anterior edge of the sternocleidomastoid muscle. Most of the injuries can be directly repaired, always having the recurrent laryngeal nerve identified to avoid any damage to it. Thoracic esophagus injuries are not common; however, they are more complex and have higher morbidity and mortality rates. Usually, they are associated with other mediastinum or thoracic lesions. The repair of those more inferior injuries consists in surgical repair with local debridement, wide drainage, primary repair, or tissue flap (muscular, pericardial, pleural, pulmonary, gastric fundus). Other procedures can be associated with the primary repair, such as esophagostomy, proximal esophageal derivation, total esophageal exclusion, gastrostomy, intraluminal tubular drainage in "T," and esophagectomy in complex cases.

Bibliography

1. Defore WW, Mattox KL, Hansen HA, et al. Surgical management of penetrating injuries of the esophagus. Am J Surg. 1997;134:734.
2. Mattox KL, et al. Injury to the esophagus, trachea, and bronchus. In: Moore EE, Mattox KL, Feliciano DV, editors. Trauma manual. 4th ed. New York: McGraw-Hill; 2003. p. 178–82.
3. Rocha AC. Trauma cervical. In: Saad Jr R, Salles RARV, Carvalho WR, Maia AM, editors. Tratado de Cirurgia do CBC. 1st ed. São Paulo: Editora Atheneu; 2009. p. 633–9.

Diaphragmatic Trauma

20

Beatriz Ortis Yazbek, Phillipe Abreu, Ana Luisa Bettega,
Zahra Farrukh Khan, and Antonio Marttos

20.1 Introduction

The diagnosis of diaphragmatic injury requires a high index of suspicion; therefore, accounting for the mechanism of trauma is crucial [1]. The most frequent causes are motor vehicle accidents and any impact force that results in raising the intraabdominal pressure with consequent diaphragmatic rupture [1]. The avulsion of the diaphragm ligaments after a lateral blow to the chest wall and its laceration by fractured ribs are also considerable mechanisms of injury [1].

The main causes of diaphragmatic injury are penetrating wounds in the thoracic-abdominal transition zone, delineated by the fourth intercostal space, sixth intercostal space laterally, and the tip of the posterior scapula and the epigastric region and the costal border inferiorly [2, 3, 4, 5].

B. O. Yazbek
Faculdade de Ciências Médicas de Santos, Santos, São Paulo, Brazil

P. Abreu (✉)
Department of Surgery, Hospital do Trabalhador Trauma Center, Federal University of Parana, Curitiba, Brazil

A. L. Bettega
Iwan Collaço Trauma Research Group, Department of Surgery, Hospital do Trabalhador Trauma Center, Federal University of Parana, Curitiba, Brazil

Z. F. Khan
Department of Surgery, University of Miami, Miller School of Medicine, Jackson Memorial Hospital, Coral Gables, FL, USA

A. Marttos
William Lehman Injury Research Center, Division of Trauma & Surgical Critical Care, Dewitt Daughtry Department of Surgery, Leonard M. Miller School of Medicine Miami, University of Miami, Miami, FL, USA

© Springer Nature Switzerland AG 2020
A. Nasr et al. (eds.), *The Trauma Golden Hour*,
https://doi.org/10.1007/978-3-030-26443-7_20

Diaphragmatic injuries lead to the equilibration of pleural and peritoneal compartment pressures creating a tendency of the viscera to migrate through the lesion into the interior of the thorax [2]. This fact can lead to a similar condition to the hypertensive pneumothorax, with potentially fatal cardiorespiratory repercussions, and cause pleural contamination by the gastrointestinal contents [2].

Injuries associated with diaphragmatic trauma are present in 75% of the cases, with lung, liver, splccn, and colon being the most injured organs and the most common harmful agent is the white weapon [2].

20.2 Types of Trauma

Blunt traumatic diaphragmatic injuries result from a rapid increase in intraabdominal pressure during an impact, causing rupture of the diaphragm. The incidence of left and right diaphragmatic hernias is similar, but when the right side lesion occurs, the mortality at the scene of the accident is greater due to the severity of the associated liver lesions.

The mortality of blunt diaphragmatic trauma is 29% due to the high energy required to cause its rupture. Morbidity is usually identified after months or years if the perforation has not been recognized and repaired initially. The evolution of these lesions includes the progressive widening of the diaphragmatic laceration, through which there may be an abdominal viscera hernia to the thorax. The lesions resulting from closed trauma are larger, varying from 5 to 10 cm, and produce herniation more easily than penetrating wounds [6, 2].

Penetrating diaphragmatic injuries are four times more common than nonpenetrating lesions and generally cause small lacerations to the right [6, 1, 7]. Therefore, most patients who suffer this type of injury mechanism do not develop immediate complications related to herniation of the abdominal organs [6, 1]. The hernia therefore develops later if the lesion is not diagnosed [1].

Classification of diaphragmatic injury is according to the American Association for the Surgery of Trauma (AAST) (depending on the size of the laceration and the amount of tissue loss) (Chart 20.1).

Chart 20.1 AAST Classification of diaphragmatic injury [6, 1, 2]

Level	Description of injury
I	Concussion
II	Laceration ≤ 2 cm
III	Laceration 2–10 cm
IV	Laceration > 10 cm with tissue loss ≤ 25 cm^2
V	Laceration with tissue loss > 25 cm^2

20.3 Symptoms

Patients presenting with diaphragmatic injuries may be asymptomatic or present a respiratory and circulatory collapse due to mass effect secondary to the presence of diaphragmatic hernia [2]. There is a wide spectrum of signs and symptoms, such as pain referred to the ipsilateral shoulder, decreased thoracic expandability, bowel sounds in thorax, abdomen excavatum, asymmetry of the right and left hypochondria, and dyspnea [2]. Clinical findings are also related to herniated viscera to the thorax, and there may be some degree of intestinal obstruction, for example [7].

20.4 Diagnosis

The diagnostic workup of this type of injury is essential to preventing the risk of development of diaphragmatic hernia with all its known complications [1, 7].

Respiratory distress initiated after blunt trauma may be indicative of abdominal viscera herniation. In this case, nasogastric tube replacement is necessary for decompression and consequent improvement of pulmonary ventilation [6]. If the hemodynamic conditions are favorable, a chest X-ray should be performed to detect signs of diaphragmatic hernia, with the presence of the nasogastric tube with contrast in the pleural space, confirming the intrathoracic stomach in which case laparotomy is indicated [6, 7].

Plain chest radiography has low accuracy for diaphragmatic lesions. Contrast examinations may show herniation from the abdominal viscera into the thorax, most commonly the stomach [2]. Findings may include elevation or blurring of the hemidiaphragm, blunting of the diaphragmatic contour, gas shadowing, and gastric probe in the thoracic projection and fluid levels if hollow viscera are herniated [6]. Chest X-ray in a simple diaphragmatic lesion without herniation would, however, be falsely negative [6].

Computed tomography of the chest and abdomen may aid in the identification of abdominal viscera in the thorax or an abnormality in the diaphragm itself, such as discontinuity, thickening, or elevation [2]. Given the difficulty of performing the diagnosis, surgical exploration can be necessary when imaging is equivocal [8].

Diaphragmatic lesions that may go unnoticed by these previously mentioned methods can be identified by endoscopic surgery, which is used in the diagnosis and treatment of lesions in hemodynamically stable patients, and can be done laparoscopically or thoracoscopically [8, 1, 2].

Once the diagnosis of a diaphragmatic lesion has been made, the presence of hemothorax and the degree of contamination of the pleural space with extravasated contents of the digestive tract should be evaluated [6, 1]. In this case, cleaning the pleural space followed by adequate drainage reduces the risks of postoperative complications [6].

Video laparoscopy is a preferred approach because it allows direct visualization of the diaphragm and peritoneal cavity, allowing diaphragm suture, reduction of herniated contents, and correction of associated abdominal viscera lesions, if present.

Video-assisted thoracoscopy allows the repair of associated diaphragmatic and thoracic lesions as well as the cleaning of the pleural cavity [2]. However, this method makes it impossible to evaluate the presence of abdominal visceral damage, which, if present, necessitates laparotomy or laparoscopy [2]. Because pulmonary complications are more frequent, diaphragmatic lesions should be approached via the abdomen when there is no other lesion requiring a thoracotomy [7].

20.5 Nonoperative Treatment

Although spontaneous healing of the diaphragm is feasible, this treatment option requires sufficient infrastructure to accurately diagnose and characterize the lesion severity and size as well as to provide long-term follow-up to ensure that the lesions do not progress and become symptomatic [2]. Based on the preliminary studies done in Murinos by Perlingeiro et al. in 2001, Gonçalves in 2008, Squeff in 2008, and Rivaben in 2009, it appears that small diaphragmatic wounds on the right side are more amenable to nonoperative management due to the protective effect of the liver in the prevention of a diaphragmatic hernia [9–11]. There are, however, no long-term studies in the national or international literature examining a series of patients who have been treated in this manner.

20.6 Operative Treatment

The repair of diaphragmatic lesions includes nonviable tissue debridement and defect closure [2]. Closure is commonly performed with interrupted "U" stitches using nonabsorbable suture in a single layer incorporating a large thickness of healthy diaphragmatic tissue [6, 1, 7]. Some surgeons advocate continuous suturing of the remaining edges of the "U" suture.

When the diaphragm is detached from the periphery, it can be reinserted into the chest wall at one to two intercostal spaces above.

Hemostasis in this layer is important because branches of the phrenic artery may be exposed at the edges of the lesion. If necessary, the pleural cavity on the side of the lesion can be drained with a multi-sealed tubular chest drain under water seal [6].

In acute cases, the primary repair should be performed by suturing [1]. In chronic cases or in the presence of a large area of lost tissue, it may be necessary to use a screen to correct hernia defects or to reconstruct with a prosthesis [1]. In addition, in chronic cases, thoracotomy is the preferred approach due to the difficulty associated with laparotomy secondary to abdominal adhesions [1].

20.7 Complications

The most common acute complications of traumatic diaphragmatic lesions are dehiscence of the suture, diaphragmatic folding due to traumatic or iatrogenic injury of the phrenic nerve, cardiorespiratory failure, hemorrhage, empyema, or subphrenic abscess [6]. Strangulated hernias, with or without perforation of abdominal viscera, and intestinal obstructions may occur as late complications [6, 1, 7].

Patients presenting with a late diagnosis of diaphragmatic hernia have a 25% mortality rate which is related to sepsis due to incarceration, ischemia, and necrosis, with potential for subsequent rupture, of the herniated abdominal viscera into the pleural space [6, 7].

The main problem stemming from diaphragmatic injury is that the negative pleuroperitoneal gradient and continuous diaphragmatic mobility prevent healing of the lesion [1]. Therefore, operative treatment is not an option [1]. Positive pressure ventilation, common in the polytraumatized patient, eradicates the gradient pleuroperitoneal; however, after improvement of the patient's clinical status and subsequent extubation may reveal, abdominal organ herniation [1–2].

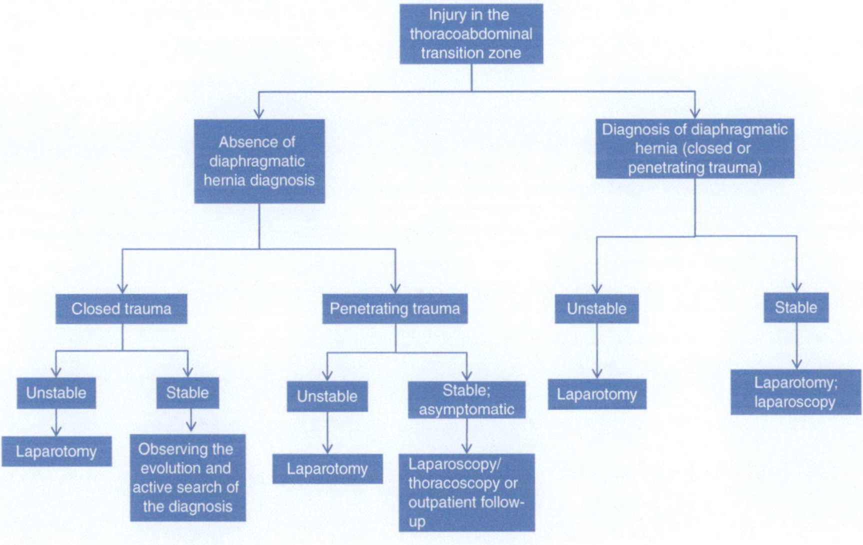

20.8 Conclusion

Trauma care surgeons are known to have a low threshold for suspecting diaphragmatic injury. Repair of this important muscle, which is fundamental to human respiration, tends to heal well with low recurrences and excellent prognosis [7]. However, unidentified and corrected lesions in this acute phase of trauma may result in minor or major complications, months or even years after the fatal trauma, thus resulting in high rates of morbidity and mortality [2].

References

1. Ribeiro MAF Jr. Fundamentals of trauma surgery. 1st ed. Rio de Janeiro: Roca; 2016.
2. Saad R Jr, et al. Treaty of surgery of CBC. 2nd ed. Atheneu: São Paulo, Rio de Janeiro, Belo Horizonte; 2015.
3. Saad JR, et al. General thoracic surgery. 2nd ed. São Paulo, Rio de Janeiro, Belo Horizonte: Atheneu; 2011.
4. Performer JAG, Saad R Jr, Lancelotti CLP, et al. Natural course of penetrating diaphragmatic injury: an experimental study in rats. Int Surg. 2007;92:1 9.
5. Zantut LF, Ivatury RR, Smith S, et al. Diagnostic and therapeutic laparoscopy and penetrating abdominal trauma: a multicenter experience. J Trauma. 1997;42:825–31.
6. Ferraz AR, et al. Clinical surgery. 1st ed. São Paulo: Manole; 2008.
7. Way LW. Surgery diagnosis and treatment. 9th ed. San Francisco: Lawrence W. Way; 1990.
8. Mattox K, et al. Treaty of surgery. 19th ed. São Paulo: Elsevier; 2015.
9. Gonçalves R. Analysis of the natural evolution of puncture wounds equivalent to 30% of the left diaphragm. Experimental study in rats. Master thesis – Santa Casa de São Paulo. São Paulo, 2008.
10. Rivaben HR. Natural history of extensive diaphragmatic wound on the right: experimental study in rats. Master thesis – Santa casa de São Paulo. São Paulo, 2011.
11. Saad JR. Should all injury of the diaphragm for penetrating injury be sutured?

Exploratory Laparotomy in Trauma

21

Marianne Reitz, Renar Brito Barros, Mariana Vieira Delazeri, Beatriz Ortis Yazbek, and Antonio Marttos

21.1 Introduction

In a patient with massive intraabdominal bleeding the feeling of distress, fear, and chaos can easily occur. However, in all of this, there is a method and art. Laparotomy in trauma is not the accelerated version of an elective surgery. It does not have to be synonymous of rusticity or inadvertent maneuvers. Time is the most important factor, but fast movements are not what will lead the surgery to success. Efficient and ordered maneuvers are what will benefit the patient.

Final conduct to these patients is the addition of an assessment that starts with the arrival of the patient in the emergency room, the findings of the exploratory laparotomy, and the interaction of the staff. Auxiliaries, nurse team, and the anesthesiologist are fundamental parts of the scenario. Exploratory laparotomy in a patient with an abdominal trauma is the higher expression of the need for organization and the development of a tactical surgical strategy. Each surgeon has his/her own

M. Reitz
Iwan Collaço Trauma Research Group, Department of Surgery, Hospital do Trabalhador Trauma Center, Federal University of Parana, Curitiba, Brazil

R. B. Barros · M. V. Delazeri
Department of Surgery, Hospital do Trabalhador Trauma Center,
Federal University of Parana, Curitiba, Brazil

B. O. Yazbek
Faculdade de Ciências Médicas de Santos, Santos, São Paulo, Brazil

A. Marttos (✉)
William Lehman Injury Research Center, Division of Trauma & Surgical Critical Care,
Dewitt Daughtry Department of Surgery, Leonard M. Miller School of Medicine Miami,
University of Miami, Miami, FL, USA
e-mail: amarttos@med.miami.edu

© Springer Nature Switzerland AG 2020
A. Nasr et al. (eds.), *The Trauma Golden Hour*,
https://doi.org/10.1007/978-3-030-26443-7_21

features; however, there is a basic line of conduct that guarantees good results with security and efficiency. Next, we propose a tactical and reproducible scheme for the execution of exploratory laparotomy in trauma.

Flowchart 1: Indications of exploratory laparotomy in blunt abdominal trauma

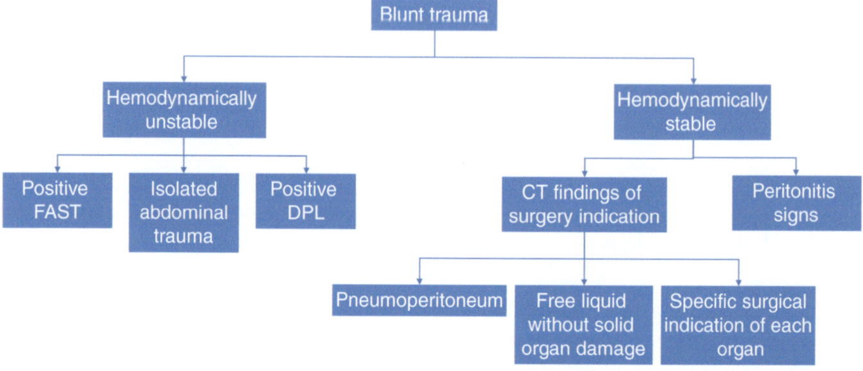

Flowchart 2: Indications of exploratory laparotomy in penetrating abdominal trauma

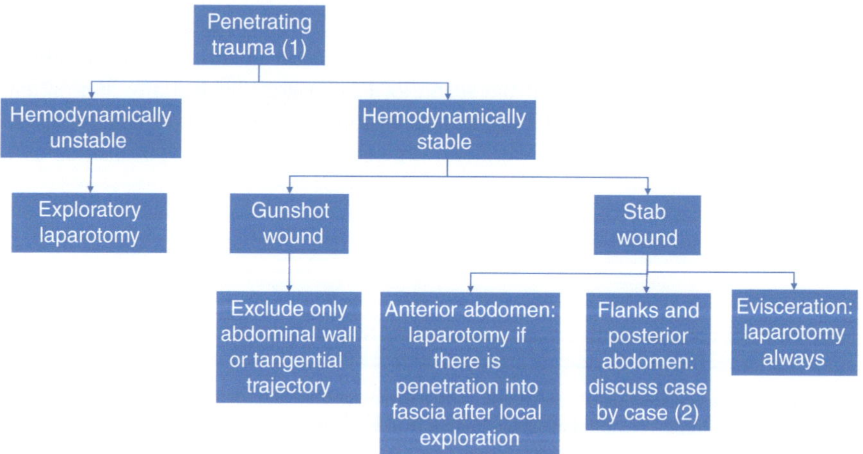

1. The nonsurgical treatment of abdominal lesions by penetrating trauma must be considered in each specific step, especially in wounds with trajectory in the right hypochondrium and retroperitoneum. To discard trajectory in the abdominal wall, a probe should be placed in the trajectory and the contrast injected. The use of this technique and computed tomography is valuable.

2. Stab wounds to the flank and posterior wall can be managed by videolaparoscopy, computed tomography, and serial clinical examination and laboratory tests. The aim is to define if there is penetration of the abdominal cavity.

Flowchart 3: Steps of the exploratory laparotomy in trauma

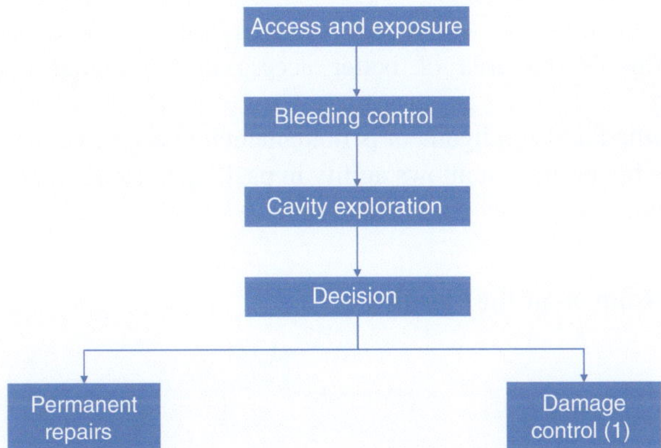

1. Damage control surgery is defined by a surgery to control the bleeding and the contamination of the cavity; it is an abbreviated laparotomy and a new surgical intervention will be required.

Flowchart 4: Access and exposition

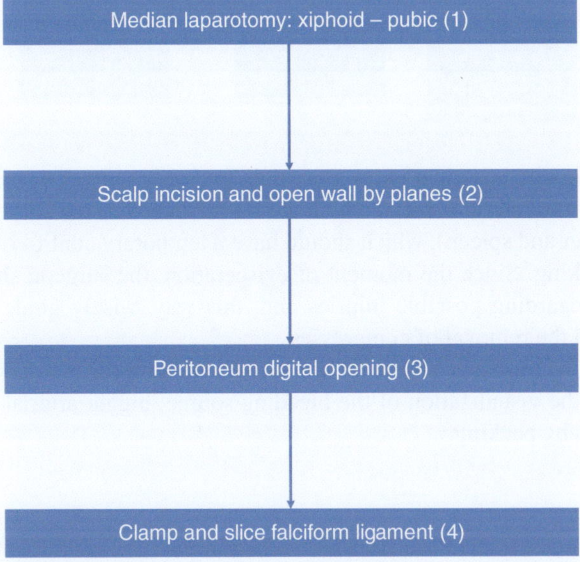

1. Patients with previous midline abdominal surgeries and a hostile abdomen can benefit from a bisubcostal incision.
2. The abdominal wall opening should be done with three scalpel movements: skin, subcutaneous tissue, and aponeurosis. Opening with a cautery is an option in hemodynamically stable patients in which the access to the cavity can be postponed.
3. Right after the umbilical scar, there is the area of greatest weakness of the peritoneum. This is the area of better access to the digital opening of the peritoneum.
4. Sectioning the falciform ligament is fundamental to access of the cavity and the depart for a better view. It allows agility in packing the supramesocolic space of the abdomen.

Flowchart 5: Control of the bleeding

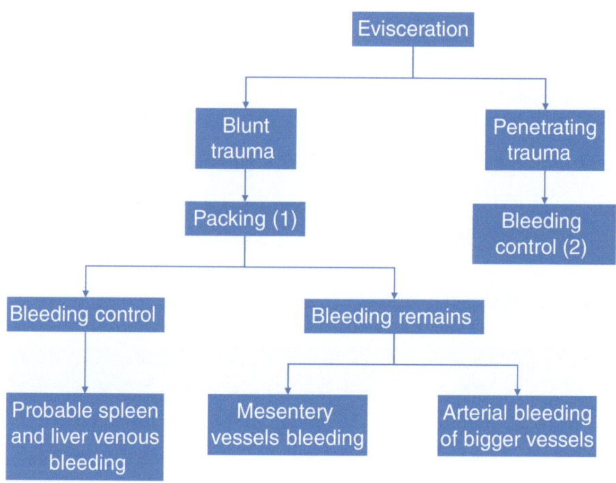

1. With eviscerated intestinal loops, two main probable sources of bleeding can be identified: mesenteric vessels, which are on the hands of the surgeon; and solid organs (liver and spleen), which should have a temporary control of the bleeding due to packing. Since the moment of evisceration, the surgeon should observe any lead regarding possible injuries and, this way, wisely guide the bleeding control and the removal of compresses.
2. In penetrating trauma, compresses are useful to remove the blood from the cavity and allow the visualization of the bleeding source; bigger arterial hemorrhages do not stop by packing.

Flowchart 6: Sequence of packing

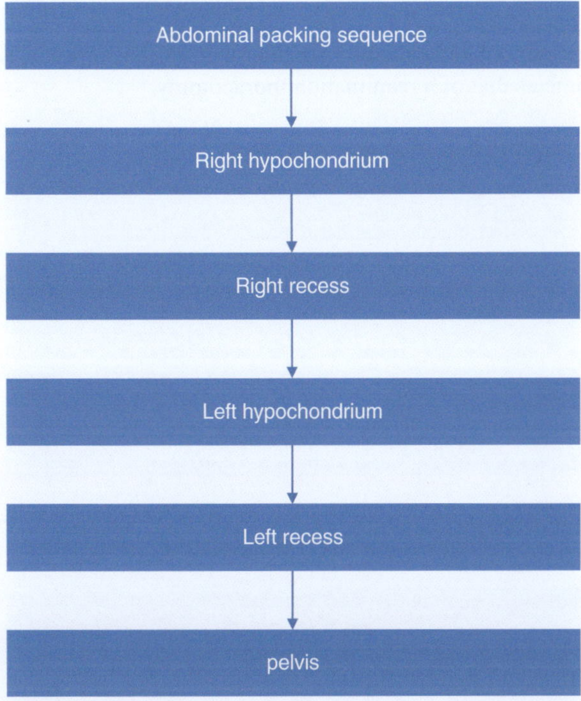

Flowchart 7: Aortic clamping

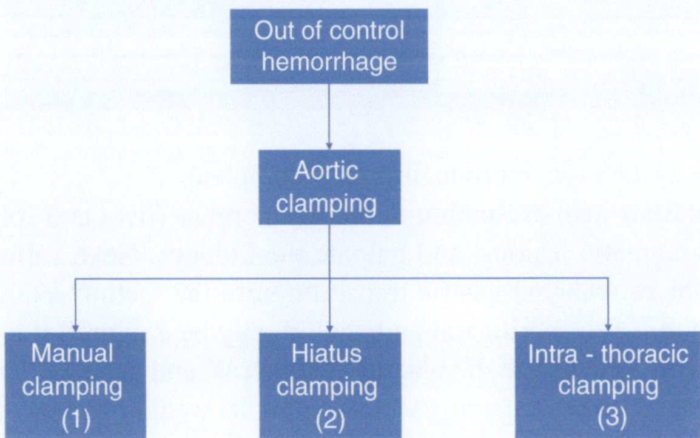

1. Clamping by the lesser omentum is easier and faster.
2. Effective clamping without needing thoracic access; complete medial peritoneal rotation is necessary.
3. Option to exsanguinated patients with imminent cardiac arrest; it is performed at the same time as that of a reanimation thoracotomy.

Flowchart 8: Exploration of abdominal cavity

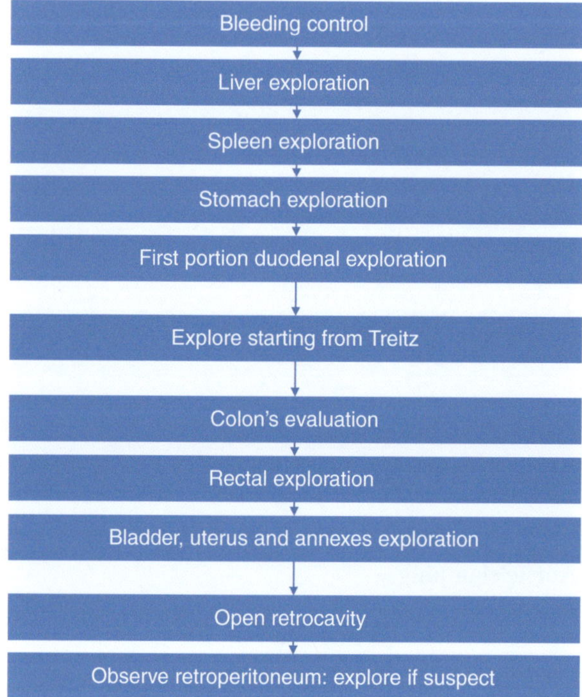

It should be systematic, reproducible, and complete.

Suggestion: Start with evaluation of the solid organs (liver and spleen), observe possible diaphragmatic lesions, and palpate the kidneys. Next, follow the hollow viscera since the esophageal-gastric transition until the rectum sequentially. Most of the duodenum is retroperitoneal and should only be explored if a lesion is suspected. In the pelvis, evaluate the bladder, the uterus, and annexes. The retrocavity should be assessed and the opening should be by its weaker area at the gastrocolic space, left to the medium line. Evaluate the posterior gastric wall and the pancreas as well.

Flowchart 9: Exploration of the retroperitoneum

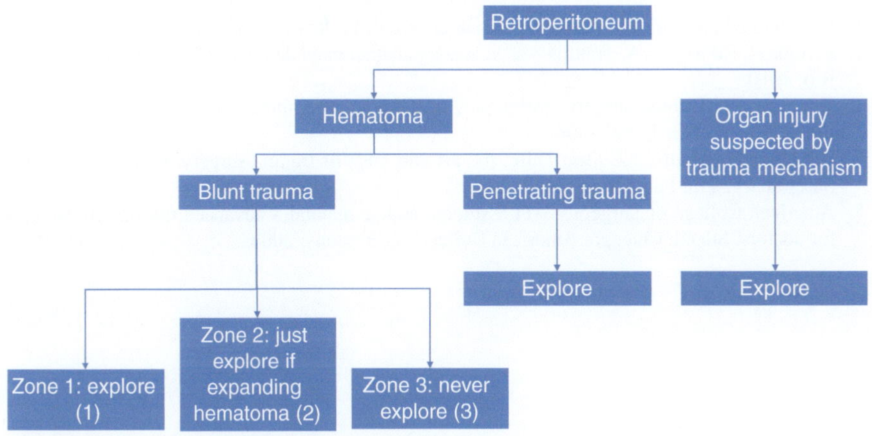

1. Zone 1: includes paravertebral area.
2. Zone 2: includes lateral hematomas.
3. Zone 3: includes hematomas at the pelvic retroperitoneum.

Flowchart 10: Definitive repair × Damage control

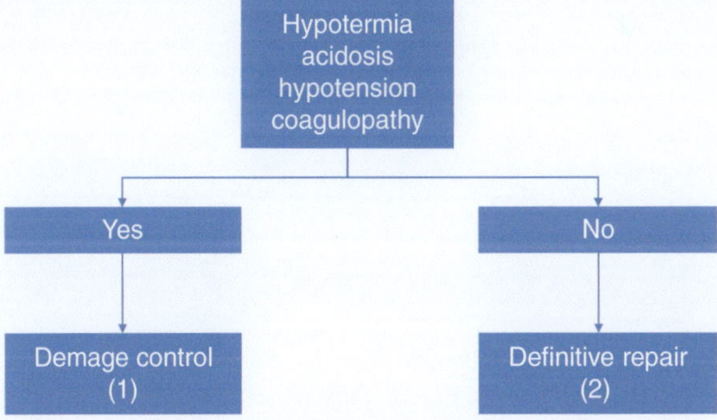

1. Damage control should be indicated before the patient enters the decline phase. Tendency of acidosis, hypotension, coagulopathy, and hypothermia trigger the process. The decision for damage control starts at the first assessment in the emergency room, or even before that, due to the information passed by the pre-hospitalar trauma life support team.
2. Definitive repair demands knowledge of the surgical treatment of each lesion on every affected organ.

Bibliography

1. Feliciano DV, Mattox KL, Moore EE Trauma. 6ª edição. Revinter; 2008.
2. Ferrada R, Rodriguez A. Trauma – sociendade panamericana de trauma. 2ª edição. ed. Atheneu Rio; 2010.
3. Donovan AJ. Trauma surgery: techniques in thoracic, abdominal, and vascular surgery. St. Louis: Mosby-Year Book; 1994.
4. Hirshberg A, Mattox KL. Top knife: the art and craft of trauma surgery. Castle Hill Barns, Shrewsbury: Tfm Publishing Ltd; 2005.
5. American College of Surgeons. ATLS student course manual – advanced trauma life support for doctors. 8th ed. Chicago: American College of Surgeons; 2008.

Blunt Abdominal Trauma

22

Denise Magalhães Machado, Eduardo Lopes Martins,
Mariana F. Jucá Moscardi, and Antonio Marttos

22.1 Introduction

Blunt abdominal trauma is frequent and the prevalence of intra-abdominal injury is 12–15% [1]. Among the main causes of death by trauma is bleeding due to abdominal organ injuries, representing 40–80% of the cases. The spleen and the liver are the organs that are more severely affected in blunt trauma, followed by the kidney [2].

Nowadays exploratory laparotomy is not the only possible treatment in trauma; it is now possible to consider conservative treatment as well. Nowadays, the nonsurgical treatment is a common strategy used in hemodynamically stable patients [2]. The cause of hemorrhagic shock in a traumatized patient is in the abdomen or thorax or pelvis. Our mission as surgeons, in blunt abdominal trauma, is to exclude the

D. M. Machado
Iwan Collaço Trauma Research Group, Department of Surgery, Hospital do Trabalhador
Trauma Center, Federal University of Parana, Curitiba, Brazil

E. L. Martins
Department of Surgery, Hospital do Trabalhador Trauma Center,
Federal University of Parana, Curitiba, Brazil

M. F. Jucá Moscardi (✉)
Telemedicine and Trauma Research, University of Miami, Ryder Trauma Center,
Miami, FL, USA

A. Marttos
William Lehman Injury Research Center, Division of Trauma & Surgical Critical Care,
Dewitt Daughtry Department of Surgery, Leonard M. Miller School of Medicine Miami,
University of Miami, Miami, FL, USA

© Springer Nature Switzerland AG 2020
A. Nasr et al. (eds.), *The Trauma Golden Hour*,
https://doi.org/10.1007/978-3-030-26443-7_22

abdomen as the source of bleeding and prove the absence of intra-abdominal surgical injuries. For the diagnosis of these two points, exams such as FAST, computed tomography, and diagnostic peritoneal lavage can be used.

Diagnostic assessment includes anamnesis, physical exam, abdominal ultrasonography (US/FAST), and/or diagnostic peritoneal lavage, computed tomography, laparotomy, and laboratory exams [1]. Remember that physical exam fails in 30% of conscious patients, because both blood and jejunal content have neutral pH and do not cause peritoneal irritation at first. Besides, in patients with a traumatic brain injury (TBI), spinal cord injury, and exogenous intoxication, physical exam cannot be performed.

Early treatment of the patients with blunt abdominal trauma depends on their hemodynamic state. Patients who do not respond to initial volume replacement are candidates to exploratory laparotomy. However, in those who present hemodynamic stability, there is a considerable variation of conduct, as demonstrated in the algorithm below [3].

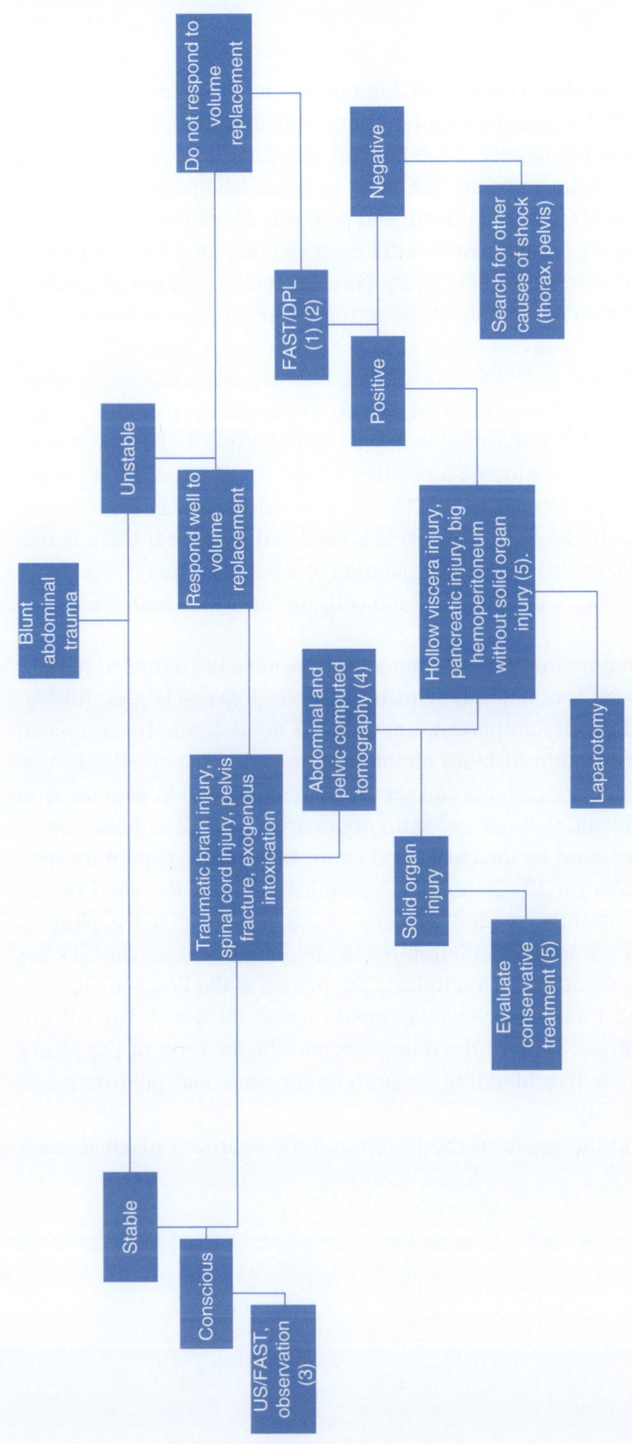
Blunt abdominal trauma
Unstable
Stable
Do not respond to volume replacement
Respond well to volume replacement
FAST/DPL (1) (2)
Negative
Positive
Search for other causes of shock (thorax, pelvis)
Hollow viscera injury, pancreatic injury, big hemoperitoneum without solid organ injury (5).
Laparotomy
Abdominal and pelvic computed tomography (4)
Traumatic brain injury, spinal cord injury, pelvis fracture, exogenous intoxication
Solid organ injury
Evaluate conservative treatment (5)
Conscious
US/FAST, observation (3)

22.2 Conclusion

1. FAST: specific ultrasound evaluation for trauma, it can be rapidly performed, with a sensibility of 90–93%, and it is not invasive. It helps the surgeon to decide for exploratory laparotomy in case of abdominal bleeding in hemodynamically unstable patients. The indications are the same as diagnostic peritoneal lavage. The disadvantage is that it does not inform you precisely about the exact site and grade of the organ injury, which justifies the need of computed tomography to evaluate the nature and extension of the injury. Besides, it is an operator-dependent exam, has limited precision to evaluate the retroperitoneum, and is less precise in obese patients [2].

2. The procedure of choice is the FAST ultrasound, because diagnostic peritoneum lavage is an invasive procedure. However, due to its simplicity, it is still a valuable feature in case FAST is not available or was inconclusive. If 10 mL or more of blood is aspirated, it is considered a positive lavage. If 10 mL of blood is not aspirated, the lavage is performed with 1000 mL of warm ringer lactate solution, followed by drainage. In this case, the test is considered positive if there is bile or plant fiber (gastric content) or in case quantitative laboratory analysis presents stained Gram bacteria, more than 100,000 red cells, or more than 500 white cells by mm^3 [4].

   For blunt abdominal trauma patients, hemoperitoneum and computed tomography showing no organ lesion, the diagnostic peritoneal lavage is a useful feature to exclude a hollow viscera perforation that was not detected by computed tomography [5]. The big trap of blunt abdominal trauma is the small intestine injury. It occurs in 2% of the patients and should be remembered in patients with free fluid on the cavity and without any solid organ injury on CT and not forgotten in patient with free fluid on the cavity and confirmed solid organ injury [6].

3. A period of observation for 12–24 hours is recommended, but the ideal period remains unknown. Currently, several authors are suggesting that the patients should be discharged without observation if the abdominal and pelvic CTs are normal and if there is no other reason to keep the patient at the hospital [1].

4. Contrasted computed tomography has a sensibility of 90–100% for spleen, liver, and kidney injuries. It gives the diagnosis and the location of the injury and shows if there is active bleeding, pseudo aneurysms, and posttraumatic arteriovenous fistulas [2].

5. Treatment depends on the grade of the lesion and the approach given to each organ.

References

1. Kendall JL, et al. Blunt abdominal trauma patients are at very low risk for intra-abdominal injury after emergency department observation. West J Emerg Med. 2011;12(4):496–504.
2. van der Vies CH, et al. Changing patterns in diagnostic strategies and the treatment of blunt injury to solid abdominal organs. Int J Emerg Med. 2011;4:47.
3. Griffin XL, Pullinger R. Are diagnostic peritoneal lavage or focused abdominal sonography for trauma safe screening investigations for hemodynamically stable patients after blunt abdominal trauma? A review of the literature. J Trauma. 2007;62:779–84.
4. Rhodes CM, Smith H, Sidwell RA. Utility and relevance of diagnostic peritoneal lavage in trauma education. J Surg Educ. 2011;68(4):313–7.
5. Wang YC, et al. Hollow organ perforation in blunt abdominal trauma: the role of diagnostic peritoneal lavage. Am J Emerg Med. 2012;30:570–3.
6. Feliciano DV, Mattox KL, Moore EF. Trauma. 6th ed. EUA: McGraw Hill; 2008.

Camila Roginski Guetter, Caroline Butler,
Guilherme Vinicius Sawczyn, Adonis Nasr, Phillipe Abreu,
Luiz Carlos Von Bahten, and Antonio Marttos

Abdominal trauma is common when evaluating a patient in a trauma setting, either in isolation or combined with other injuries. According to the National Trauma Data Bank, the incidence surpasses 90,000 cases in 2013, with a 12.8% mortality rate. Abdominal trauma is classified according to mechanism, either blunt or penetrating, and each demonstrates different patterns of injury that dictate pathways for evaluation and management. In this chapter, we focus on the evaluation and management of penetrating abdominal trauma.

23.1 Introduction

Historically, penetrating abdominal trauma would prompt mandatory exploratory laparotomy. However, unacceptably high rates of negative or nontherapeutic laparotomy have led to a change in practice. Incidence of unnecessary laparotomy is reported to range from 23% to 53% for abdominal stab wounds (SWs), and from 5.3% to 27% for abdominal gunshot wounds (GSWs). Complications following

C. R. Guetter · G. V. Sawczyn · A. Nasr · P. Abreu (⊠)
Iwan Collaço Trauma Research Group, Department of Surgery, Hospital do Trabalhador Trauma Center, Federal University of Parana, Curitiba, Brazil

C. Butler
Ryder Trauma Center – Jackson Health System, Miller School of Medicine, University of Miami, Miami, FL, USA

L. C. Von Bahten
Department of Surgery, Hospital do Trabalhador Trauma Center,
Federal University of Parana, Curitiba, Brazil

A. Marttos
William Lehman Injury Research Center, Division of Trauma & Surgical Critical Care, Dewitt Daughtry Department of Surgery, Leonard M. Miller School of Medicine Miami, University of Miami, Miami, FL, USA

© Springer Nature Switzerland AG 2020
A. Nasr et al. (eds.), *The Trauma Golden Hour*,
https://doi.org/10.1007/978-3-030-26443-7_23

nontherapeutic laparotomy are well documented and include small bowel obstructions, ileus, wound infection, pneumonia, aspiration, complications from anesthesia, and increased hospital length of stay. Additionally, advancements in imaging modalities and other diagnostic tools, as well as the success of nonoperative management (NOM) of certain solid organ injuries, mean that fewer patients are now taken to the operating room in a mandatory fashion following penetrating abdominal trauma. While immediate laparotomy is still indicated for patients who present with hemodynamic instability, signs of shock, evisceration, impalement, or peritonitis, further investigation and/or serial clinical examinations can be undertaken in the stable patient without evidence of peritonitis. It is important to note that a prerequisite of NOM is an awake and examinable patient with a reliable abdominal exam. Head injury, high spinal cord injury, depressed mental status due to intoxication, sedation, or anesthesia all mandate further diagnostic investigation or laparotomy to exclude intraperitoneal injury.

Among different mechanisms of penetrating abdominal trauma, stab wounds (SWs) occur more frequently, whereas gunshot wounds (GSWs) are associated with higher mortality rates and more severe injury patterns due to the greater energy and cavitation created by the projectile's path. While the NOM of abdominal stab wounds is well established, abdominal gunshot wounds have higher rates of intraperitoneal injury and therefore more often require laparotomy. However, the clinical presentation of the patient, location of injury, and index of suspicion for peritoneal violation are considered in the evaluation and management algorithms for both stab wounds and gunshot wounds to the abdomen.

23.2   Abdominal Gunshot Wounds (GSWs)

Exploratory laparotomy is mandatory in cases of abdominal GSW with evidence of evisceration, peritonitis, and/or hemodynamic instability. Plain radiography prior to proceeding to the operating room, if the patient is not in extremis, may help determine the path and number of projectiles.

In cases in which there is no immediate indication for surgery (Table 23.1), isolated right upper quadrant injury in a hemodynamically stable patient, or a suspected tangential bullet tract, patients should undergo further evaluation with imaging. The entrance and exit wounds, if present, should be identified with radiopaque markers and chest and abdominal X-rays taken in order to identify the location of the ballistic. If a bullet is identified on an anterior-posterior projection,

Table 23.1 Absolute indications for exploratory laparotomy in abdominal GSW

1. Hemodynamic instability
2. Peritonitis
3. Evisceration
4. Unreliable physical examination, depressed GCS, or associated neurologic injury

Abbreviations: *GSW* gunshot wound, *GCS* Glasgow coma scale
Ref: The authors

cross-table lateral films can help in further localizing it. If the patient remains hemodynamically normal and without signs of peritonitis, the clinician should strongly consider computed tomography (CT) with intravenous contrast.

The main goal of CT scan is tract delineation and identification of intraperitoneal injuries. A high-quality CT scan may identify an entirely extraperitoneal tract or a solid organ injury (e.g., liver, kidney, spleen), that can be managed nonoperatively in the stable patient. Conversely, CT signs of hollow viscous injury such as pneumoperitoneum or free fluid in the absence of solid organ injury should prompt laparotomy.

Navsaria et al. [4] performed a prospective study of selective CT scanning in 1106 patients presenting with a GSW to the abdomen. Immediate laparotomy was performed in 75.4% of patients, of which 3.5% was deemed unnecessary based on intraoperative findings. Nonoperative management was performed in 24.6% of patients, 30.1% of whom were managed with serial examination alone, and 69.9% with CT scan and serial examination. Indications for CT scan were a RUQ or right thoracoabdominal trajectory, hematuria, and/or trajectory concerns by the surgeon. With this strategy, they reported a 95.2% success rate of nonoperative management. All of those patients who failed NOM developed increasing abdominal tenderness. The study concluded that clinical examination is critical and accurate in identifying patients who require immediate laparotomy after abdominal GSW, and that selective use of CT scanning is safe and efficient.

Patients undergoing NOM should be closely monitored and kept NPO. Serial clinical examinations should be performed ideally by an experienced clinician and the same team. Hemoglobin levels should be monitored every 4–6 hours. If the patient at any point develops hemodynamic instability and/or peritonitis, laparotomy is then indicated. However, if the patient's clinical condition improves, diet should be advanced after 24 hours of observation and, if well tolerated, the patient may be transferred to the floor or discharged home, depending on the clinical circumstance (Fig. 23.1).

23.3 Abdominal Stab Wounds

Similar to abdominal gunshot wounds, immediate exploratory laparotomy is indicated for patients with abdominal SW who present with hemodynamic instability, evisceration, peritonitis, or impalement.

In hemodynamically stable, asymptomatic patients with an SW to the anterior abdominal wall, defined as the area between the costal margin, the anterior axillary lines, and the inguinal ligaments, local wound exploration can be performed. If penetration of the anterior rectus sheath is definitively excluded, the abdominal wound can be closed and the patient discharged home. If local wound exploration identifies penetration of the anterior rectus sheath, or if the entirety of the tract and the fascia are not clearly visualized, particularly in obese patients and in those with tangential wounds tracking through multiple muscle layers, the patient should either undergo serial clinical examination, or further diagnostic investigation should considered.

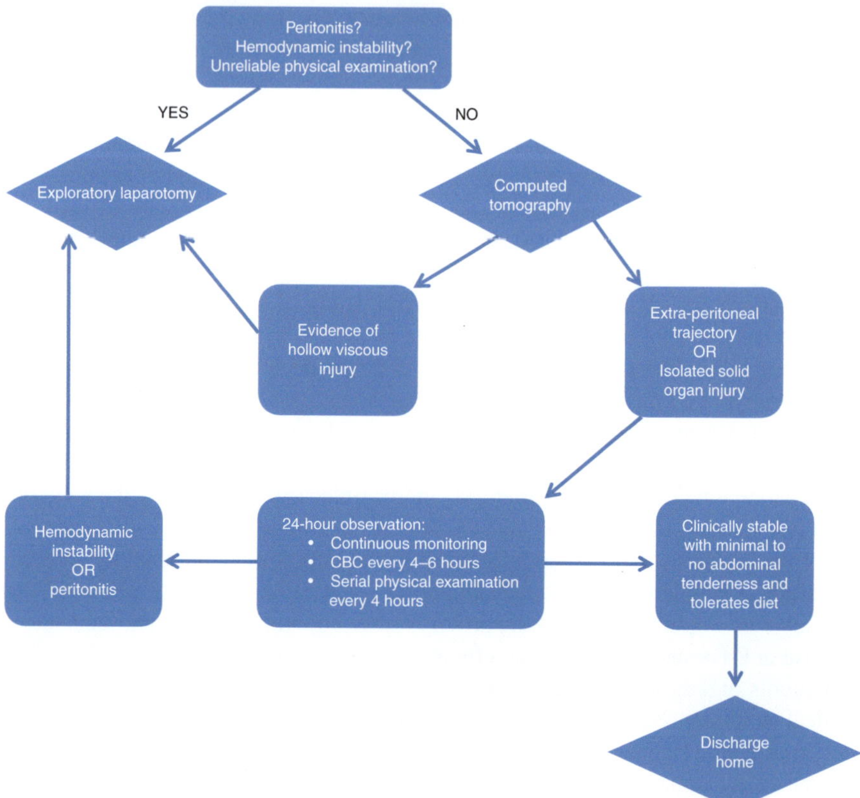

Fig. 23.1 Abdominal gunshot wounds

The role of diagnostic laparoscopy for detection of peritoneal violation remains unclear. Violation of the peritoneum does not necessarily indicate intraperitoneal injury, and therefore this technique may still lead to a high rate of unnecessary laparotomy. Fabian et al. [7] examined the use of diagnostic laparoscopy (DL) in trauma. DL was performed following positive local wound exploration. For patients with stab wounds to the anterior abdomen and positive LWE, no peritoneal penetration was detected at DL in 49%. Of the 51% with peritoneal penetration who then underwent laparotomy, 31% were therapeutic, 6% were nontherapeutic, and 13% were negative. Therefore, while DL is sensitive for detection of peritoneal penetration, it is less sensitive for intraperitoneal injury requiring laparotomy, and therefore is not routinely recommended. The most common use of DL in trauma is in the setting of left-sided penetrating thoracoabdominal trauma in order to evaluate for diaphragmatic injury.

Therefore, when local wound exploration is positive for fascial or peritoneal penetration in an asymptomatic patient, serial clinical examination should be performed. Should the patient develop hemodynamic instability or signs of peritonitis, laparotomy should be performed expeditiously. If the patient remains clinically stable with minimal to no abdominal tenderness after 24 hours of observation, patients may be discharged home after satisfactory diet toleration with a plan of follow-up in the outpatient setting.

Finally, in contrast to anterior abdominal stab wounds, stab wounds to the flank and back typically will not present with signs of peritonitis. CT scan with IV contrast is indicated in patients presenting with penetrating trauma to the flank or back in order to evaluate for retroperitoneal injury. Signs of colonic injury or small bowel (Table 23.2) should prompt laparotomy. Solid organ injuries in the hemodynamically stable patient may be managed nonoperatively with serial clinical examinations as per the above algorithms (Fig. 23.2).

Table 23.2 AAST small bowel injury severity scale

Grade	Type of injury	Description of Injury
I	Hematoma	Contusion or hematoma without devascularization
	Laceration	Partial thickness, no perforation
II	Laceration	Laceration < 50% circumference
III	Laceration	Laceration ≥ 50% circumference
IV	Laceration	Transection of the small bowel
V	Laceration	Transection of the small bowel with segmental tissue loss
	Vascular	Devascularized segment

Remarks: Advance one grade for multiple injuries up to grade III
Abbreviation: *AAST* American Association for the Surgery of Trauma
Ref: [9]

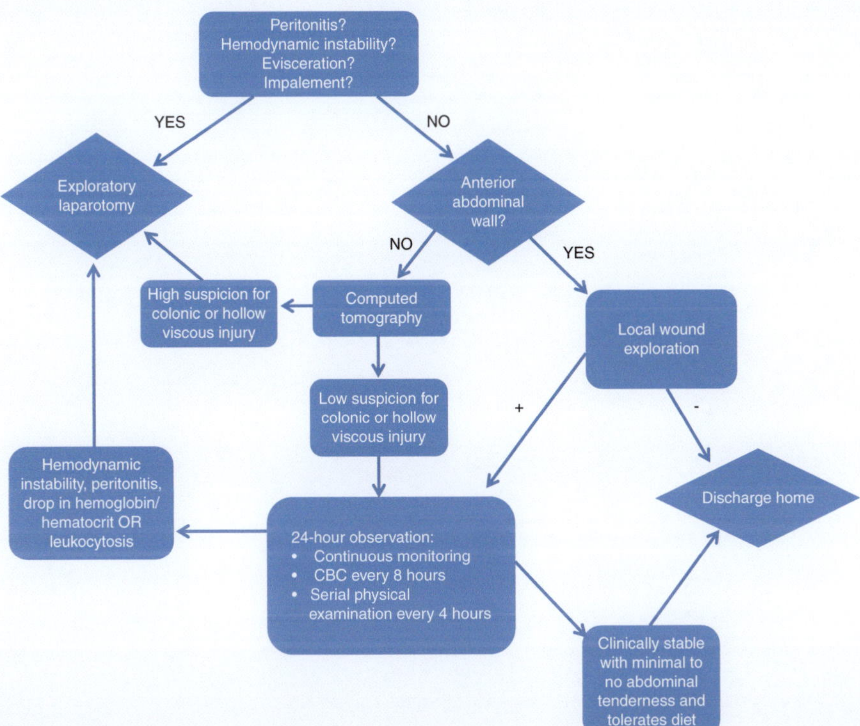

Fig. 23.2 Abdominal stab wounds [1–3, 5, 6, 8]

References

1. Biffl WL, Kaups KL, Cothren CC, et al. Management of patients with anterior abdominal stab wound: a Western Trauma Association multicenter trial. J Trauma. 2009;66(5):1294–301.
2. Biffl WL, Kaups KL, Cothren CC, et al. Validating the western trauma association algorithm for managing patients with anterior abdominal stab wounds: a Western Trauma Association multicenter trial. J Trauma. 2011;71(6):1494–502.
3. Committee on Trauma. American College of Surgeons: National Trauma Data Bank annual report 2014. Chicago: American College of Surgeons; 2014.
4. Navsaria PH, Nicol AJ, Edu S, Ganhi R, Ball CG. Selective nonoperative management in 1106 patients with abdominal gunshot wounds: conclusions on safety, efficacy, and the role of selective CT imaging in a prospective single-center study. Ann Surg. 2015;261(4):760–4.
5. Puskarich MA. Initial evaluation and management of abdominal gunshot wounds in adults. Uptodate.com; 2015
6. Townsend CM. Sabiston textbook of surgery: the biological basis of modern surgical practice. 19th ed. Texas: Elsevier Saunders; 2012.
7. Fabian TC, Croce MA, Stewart RM, Prtichard FE, Minard G, Kudsk KA. A prospective analysis of diagnostic laparoscopy in trauma. Ann Surg. 1993;217(5):557–64.
8. Como JJ, Bokhari F, Chiu WC, Duane TM, Holevar MR, Tandoh MA, Ivatury RR, Scalea TM. Practice management guidelines for selective nonoperative management of penetrating abdominal trauma. J Trauma. 2010;68(3):721–33.
9. Weinberg JA, Croce MA. Penetrating injuries to the stomach, duodenum, and small bowel. Curr Trauma Rep. 2015;1:107–12.

Liver and Bile Duct Trauma

24

Ana Gabriela Clemente, Silvania Klug Pimentel,
Mariana F. Jucá Moscardi, Jonathan Meizoso,
and Rishi Rattan

24.1 Introduction

Management of blunt hepatic trauma has evolved significantly over the last twenty years, with nonoperative management being the primary strategy in over 80% of cases. This has resulted in decreased incidence of morbidity and mortality.

In all cases, management strategy is dictated by the patient's physical examination, hemodynamic status, and diagnostic imaging results. Hemodynamically unstable patients and/or those with evidence of intra-abdominal free fluid require laparotomy. Stable patients can be deferred to CT scan for further imaging workup, with the majority only requiring ICU admission and nonoperative management. Delayed complications, including hemorrhage, abscess, and biliary fistula, can often be managed with minimally invasive and/or interventional radiologic techniques.

Intrahepatic bile duct injuries are always related to liver trauma and is approached in the same way. Extrahepatic bile duct injuries are usually related to other organ

A. G. Clemente
Iwan Collaço Trauma Research Group, Department of Surgery, Hospital do Trabalhador
Trauma Center, Federal University of Parana, Curitiba, Brazil

S. K. Pimentel
Department of Surgery, Hospital do Trabalhador Trauma Center,
Federal University of Parana, Curitiba, Brazil

M. F. Jucá Moscardi (⊠)
Telemedicine and Trauma Research, University of Miami, Ryder Trauma Center,
Miami, FL, USA

J. Meizoso
Ryder Trauma Center – Jackson Health System, Miami, FL, USA

Miller School of Medicine, University of Miami, Miami, FL, USA

R. Rattan
Division of Trauma Surgery & Critical Care, DeWitt Daughtry Family Department of
Surgery, Miller School of Medicine, University of Miami, Miami, FL, USA

© Springer Nature Switzerland AG 2020
A. Nasr et al. (eds.), *The Trauma Golden Hour*,
https://doi.org/10.1007/978-3-030-26443-7_24

involvement and are surgically managed by primary reconstruction or drainage followed by elective reconstruction.

Gall bladder injury requires cholecystectomy as surgical treatment.

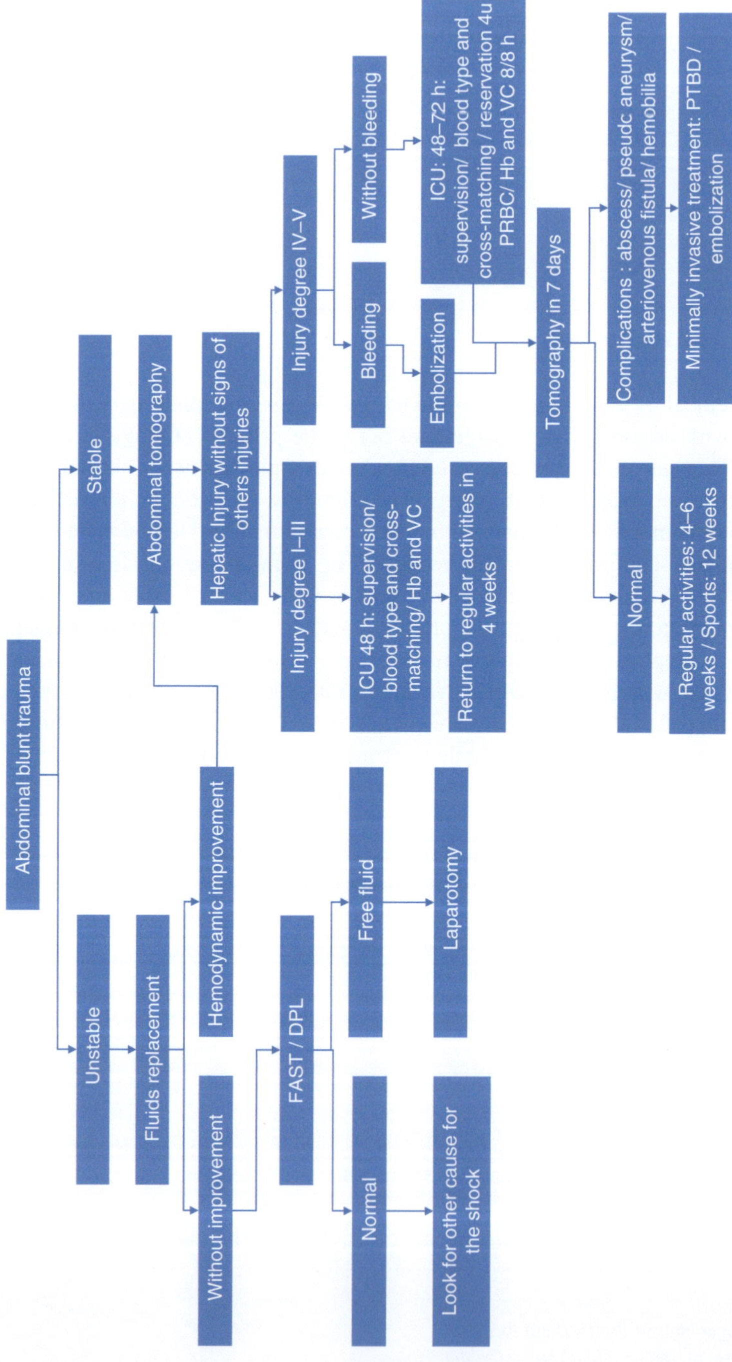

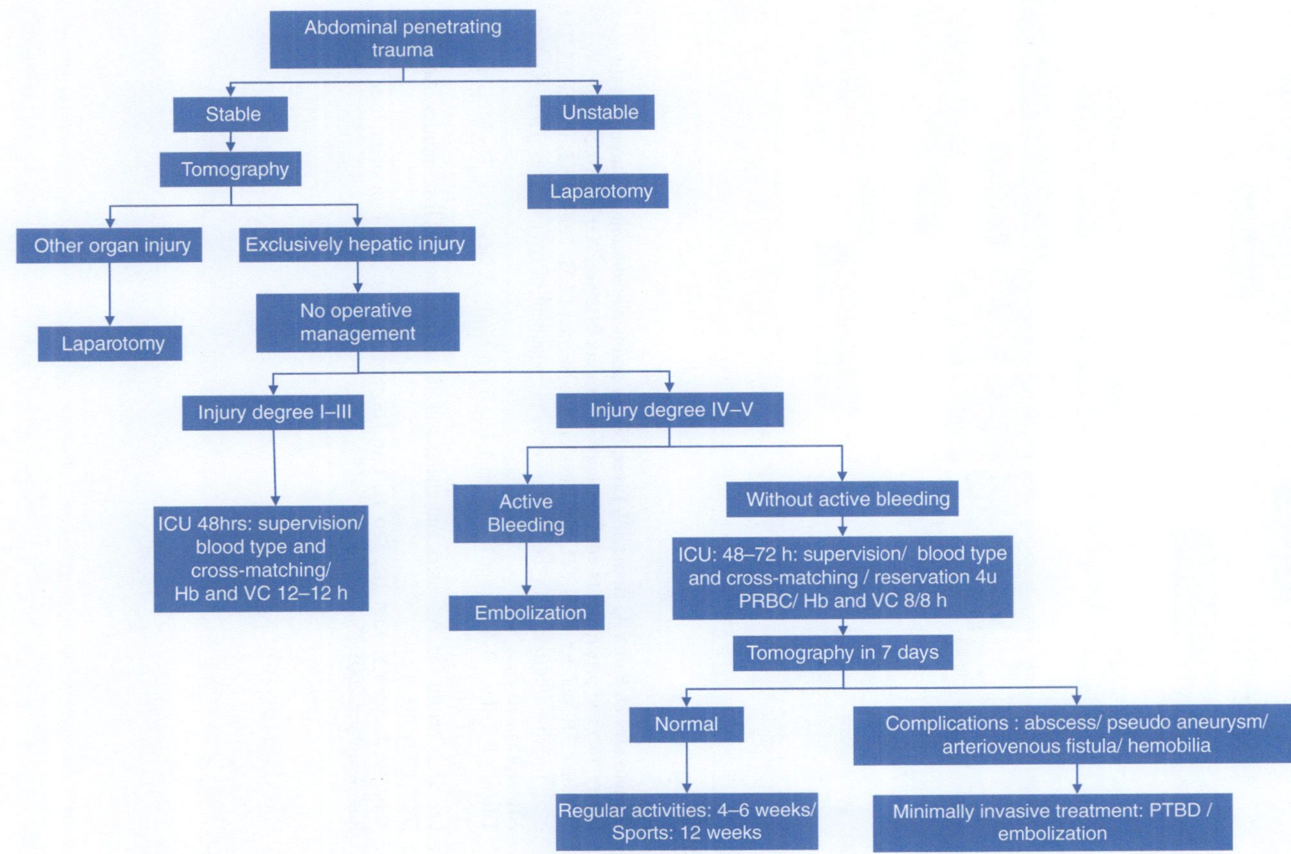

Abdominal penetrating trauma
Stable
Unstable
Tomography
Laparotomy
Other organ injury
Exclusively hepatic injury
Laparotomy
No operative management
Injury degree I–III
Injury degree IV–V
ICU 48hrs: supervision/ blood type and cross-matching/ Hb and VC 12–12 h
Active Bleeding
Without active bleeding
Embolization
ICU: 48–72 h: supervision/ blood type and cross-matching / reservation 4u PRBC/ Hb and VC 8/8 h
Tomography in 7 days
Normal
Complications : abscess/ pseudo aneurysm/ arteriovenous fistula/ hemobilia
Regular activities: 4–6 weeks/ Sports: 12 weeks
Minimally invasive treatment: PTBD / embolization

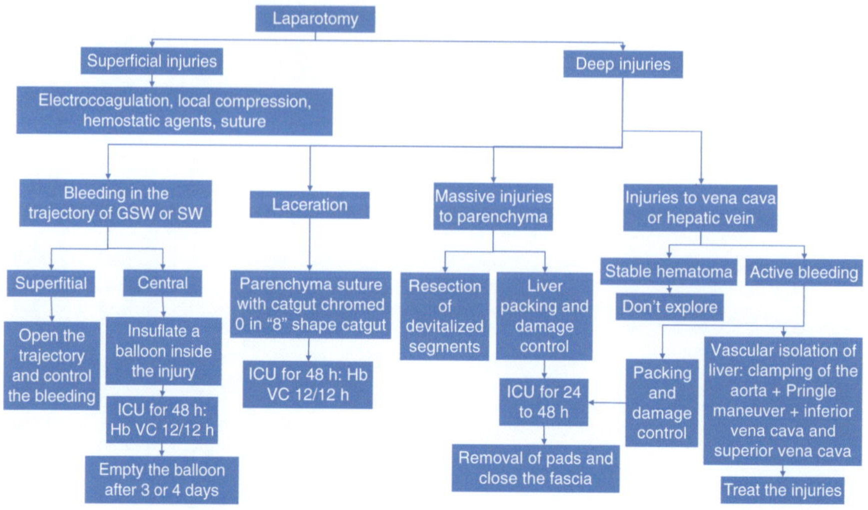

Bibliography

1. Demetriades D, Salim A, Berne TV. Liver, biliary and pancreatic injury. Surgery of the liver, biliary tract and pancreas. 4th ed. Philadelphia: Sauders Elsevier; 2007. p. 1035–48.
2. Saltzherr TP, van der Vlies CH, van Lienden KP, Beenen LFM, Ponsen KJ, van Gulik TM, et al. Improved outcomes in the non-operative management of liver injuries. HPB (Oxford). 2011;13(5):350–5.
3. Timothy F, Tiffany B. Liver and biliary tract. In: Trauma. 6th ed. New York: The McGraw-Hill; 2008. p. 637–60.
4. Lee SK, Carrillo EH. Advances and changes in the management of liver injuries. Am Surg. 2007;73(3):201–6.
5. Yoon W, Jeong YY, Kim JK, Seo JJ, Lim HS, Shin SS, et al. CT in blunt liver trauma. Radiographics. 2005;25(1):87–104.

Blunt Splenic Trauma

25

Jéssica Romanelli Amorim de Souza,
Mariana F. Jucá Moscardi, Phillipe Abreu,
Thiago Américo Murakami, Fábio Henrique de Carvalho,
and Gerrard Daniel Pust

25.1 Introduction

Spleen injury is one of the most common injuries of abdominal trauma after liver and kidneys injuries and is the most common organ injured on blunt abdominal trauma, representing between 30% and 50% off all abdominal solid organ injuries.

Spleen injury should be recognized as quickly as possible to prevent the patient bleed to death. Treatment of spleen injury has changed a lot in the last few years, increasing the number of nonoperative management. However, 40% of all spleen injury still needs immediate operative intervention.

There are some criteria to define patients who can be managed nonoperatively. The first criterion is hemodynamic stability; patients with hypotension (systolic

J. R. A. de Souza · P. Abreu · T. A. Murakami
Iwan Collaço Trauma Research Group, Department of Surgery, Hospital do Trabalhador Trauma Center, Federal University of Parana, Curitiba, Brazil

M. F. Jucá Moscardi (✉)
Telemedicine and Trauma Research, University of Miami, Ryder Trauma Center, Miami, FL, USA

F. H. de Carvalho
Department of Surgery, Hospital do Trabalhador Trauma Center, Federal University of Parana, Curitiba, Brazil

G. D. Pust
Division of Trauma Surgery & Critical Care, DeWitt Daughtry Family Department of Surgery, Miller School of Medicine, University of Miami, Miami, FL, USA

© Springer Nature Switzerland AG 2020
A. Nasr et al. (eds.), *The Trauma Golden Hour*,
https://doi.org/10.1007/978-3-030-26443-7_25

blood pressure <90 mmHg) should undergo ultrasonography called FAST or DPA, to identify any intra-abdominal fluids. If FAST or DPA is positive, the patient should be taken immediately to operation room for exploratory laparotomy. Patients with no hypotension and who are hemodynamically stable are candidates for abdominal CT scan with intravenous contrast to define the best treatment.

The second important criterion is the presence of peritonitis; if the patient is stable but peritonitis is present, operative treatment should be considered.

Patient with hemodynamic stability and without signs of peritonitis should undergo CT scan. Angiography should be considered if CT scan shows splenic injury greater than III, presence of contrast blush, aneurysm, or arteriovenous fistula, moderate hemoperitoneum, or another evidence of ongoing splenic bleeding. If none of these signs and no other severe injury are present, nonoperative management can be preferred.

Nonoperative management should only be considered in a hospital with capabilities for continual monitoring, serial clinical evaluations, and an operating room available for urgent laparotomy.

Once nonoperative management is chosen, some best measures should be taken. The patient must be kept monitored in the first 48 hours and daily blood count should be considered on the first 4 days. New CT scan or arteriography exam should be considered if patient presents persistent systemic inflammatory response, increasing/persistent abdominal pain, and unexplained drop in hemoglobin. If new instability shows up, the patient should undergo exploratory laparotomy.

There is no consensus about another routine CT after nonoperative management of blunt splenic injury.

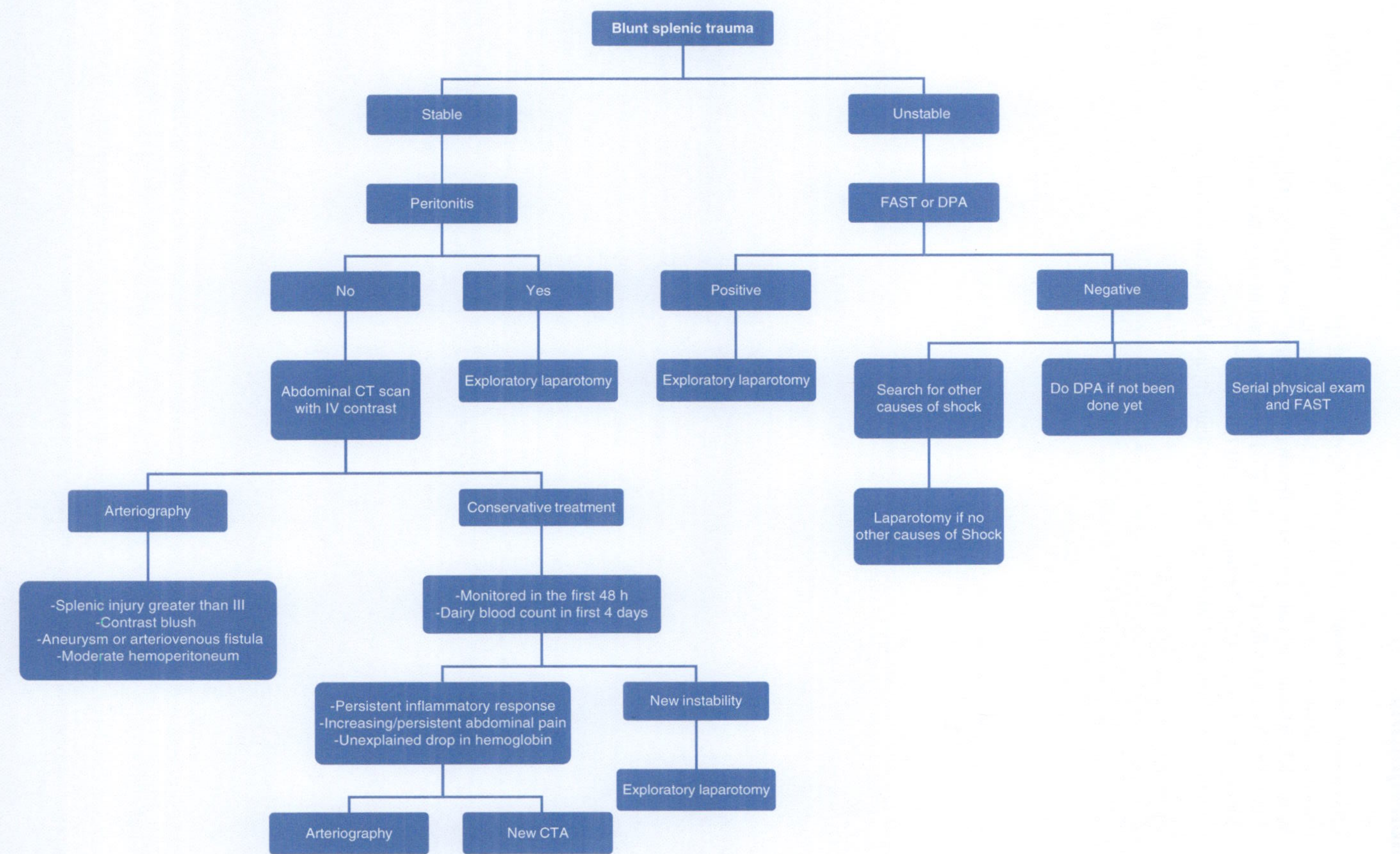

Blunt splenic trauma
Stable
Unstable
Peritonitis
FAST or DPA
No
Yes
Positive
Negative
Abdominal CT scan with IV contrast
Exploratory laparotomy
Exploratory laparotomy
Search for other causes of shock
Do DPA if not been done yet
Serial physical exam and FAST
Laparotomy if no other causes of Shock
Arteriography
Conservative treatment
-Splenic injury greater than III
-Contrast blush
-Aneurysm or arteriovenous fistula
-Moderate hemoperitoneum
-Monitored in the first 48 h
-Dairy blood count in first 4 days
-Persistent inflammatory response
-Increasing/persistent abdominal pain
-Unexplained drop in hemoglobin
New instability
Exploratory laparotomy
Arteriography
New CTA

Bibliography

1. El-Matbouly M, Jabbour G, El-Menyar A, et al. Blunt splenic trauma: assessment, management and outcomes. Surgeon. 2016;14(1):52–8. Elsevier Ltd.
2. Matox KL, Moore EE, Feliciano DV. Trauma, 7th edition. New York: McGraw Hill; 2013.
3. Olthof DC, Van der Vlies CH, Goslings JC. Evidence-based management and controversies in blunt splenic trauma. Curr Trauma Rep. 2017;3(1):32–7.
4. Yorkgitis BK. Primary Care of the Blunt Splenic Injured Adult. Am J Med. 2017;130(3):365. e1–5.

Gastric Injuries

26

Ana Luisa Bettega, Fernanda Cristina Silva,
Gustavo Rodrigues Alves Castro,
Emanuel Antonio Grasselli, Beatriz Ortis Yazbek,
Anthony Ferrantella, and Antonio Marttos

26.1 Introduction

Gastric injuries are common in penetrating trauma to the abdomen and lower chest, but in blunt trauma, they are rare and account for a small minority of hollow viscus injuries. Although gastric injuries caused by penetrating trauma are not life threatening during the so-called golden hour, associated thoracic and vascular injuries can compromise the hemodynamic status of the patient. Therefore, initial management of the patient should follow the priority principles established by ATLS.

Like injuries to other hollow viscera, gastric injuries caused by blunt abdominal trauma can manifest late, making the diagnosis more difficult and the prognosis worse. Leakage of stomach contents causes signs of peritoneal irritation on physical exam. This finding in the setting of an appropriate mechanism of trauma is the key to maintaining a high index of suspicion for gastric injuries. Diagnostic peritoneal lavage, abdominal ultrasound (FAST), and computed tomography may be used to

A. L. Bettega (✉) · E. A. Grasselli
Iwan Collaço Trauma Research Group, Department of Surgery, Hospital do Trabalhador Trauma Center, Federal University of Parana, Curitiba, Brazil

F. C. Silva · G. R. A. Castro
Department of Surgery, Hospital do Trabalhador Trauma Center, Federal University of Parana, Curitiba, Brazil

B. O. Yazbek
Faculdade de Ciências Médicas de Santos, Santos, São Paulo, Brazil

A. Ferrantella
Department of Surgery, University of Miami, Miami, FL, USA

A. Marttos
William Lehman Injury Research Center, Division of Trauma & Surgical Critical Care, Dewitt Daughtry Department of Surgery, Leonard M. Miller School of Medicine Miami, University of Miami, Miami, FL, USA

© Springer Nature Switzerland AG 2020
A. Nasr et al. (eds.), *The Trauma Golden Hour*,
https://doi.org/10.1007/978-3-030-26443-7_26

141

help guide the diagnosis. Other findings can suggest the diagnosis such as the presence of a pneumoperitoneum on plain X-ray or bloody aspirate upon nasogastric tube placement. The mechanism of injury, physical exam, and diagnostic imaging can suggest gastric injuries; however, the gold standard remains exploratory laparotomy.

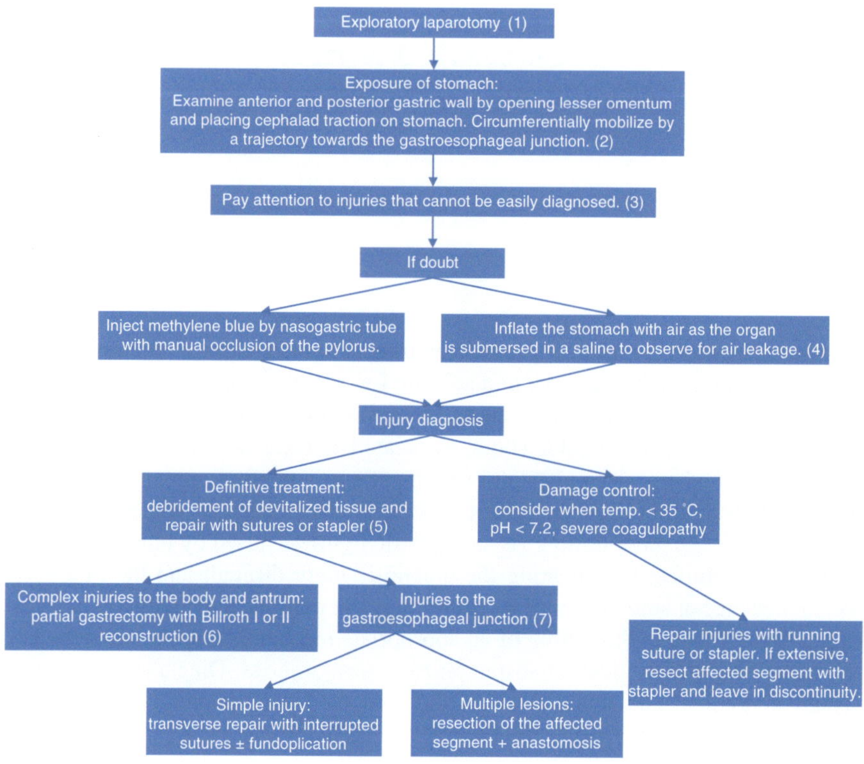

26.2 Conclusion

(1) Priority should be given to controlling active hemorrhage and containing gross contamination within the abdominal cavity.

(2) Nasogastric tube decompression can facilitate mobilization of the stomach. Consider ligation of the short gastric vessels to facilitate mobilization of the gastric fundus and avoid iatrogenic injury to the spleen. Traction of the left hepatic lobe may facilitate the exposure.

(3) Injuries to the posterior wall of the gastric fundus and lesser curvature may not be readily apparent.

(4) If air leakage is observed but no injury is found, an intraoperative endoscopy should be performed in the hemodynamically stable patient.

(5) Full-thickness sutures should be placed to ensure adequate hemostasis. Tangential wounds may be treated by resection and repair with suture or stapler. Sutures placed near the pylorus require special attention due to the risk of stenosis. Consider pyloroplasty with transverse closure.

(6) The aim is to control the bleeding and re-establish continuity.

(7) For simple stab wounds in the anterior esophageal wall, repair with transverse interrupted sutures. Partial fundoplication can also be considered. When there are several injuries, resect the affected segment and proceed with anastomosis.

Bibliography

1. Velmahos GC, Degiannis E, Doll D. Penetrating trauma. 2nd ed. Berlin Heidelberg: Springer-Verlag; 2017.
2. Mattox KL, Feliciano DV, Moore EE. Trauma. 8th ed. New York: McGraw-Hill Education; 2017.
3. Asensio JA, Trunkey DD. Therapy of trauma surgical critical care. 2nd ed. Philadelphia: Elsevier; 2016.

Small Bowel Injuries

27

Leonardo Lasari Melo, Renato Vianna Soares,
Alexandre Vianna Soares, Regina Maria Goolkate,
Maymoona Attiyat, and Antonio Marttos

27.1 Introduction

The small intestine is divided into three parts with different functions and anatomy: duodenum, jejunum, and ileum.

The duodenojejunal transition happens at the level of the ligament of Treitz, which marks the duodenojejunal junction. The jejunum comprises 40% of the small intestine. The transition between jejunum and ileum is not usually well defined. The entirety of the small intestine in an adult measures about 6 m. It is especially important to distinguish between jejunal and ileal resection especially in cases of extensive bowel resection, as the ileum is important for the absorption of specific nutrients like Vitamin B12 and bile salts. Also, the density of bacterial population increases as you move distally in the small intestine.

L. L. Melo · R. M. Goolkate
Iwan Collaço Trauma Research Group, Department of Surgery, Hospital do Trabalhador Trauma Center, Federal University of Parana, Curitiba, Brazil

R. V. Soares · A. V. Soares
Department of Surgery, Hospital do Trabalhador Trauma Center, Federal University of Parana, Curitiba, Brazil

M. Attiyat
Ryder Trauma Center – Jackson Health System, Miller School of Medicine, University of Miami, Miami, FL, USA

A. Marttos (✉)
William Lehman Injury Research Center, Division of Trauma & Surgical Critical Care, Dewitt Daughtry Department of Surgery, Leonard M. Miller School of Medicine Miami, University of Miami, Miami, FL, USA
e-mail: amarttos@med.miami.edu

© Springer Nature Switzerland AG 2020
A. Nasr et al. (eds.), *The Trauma Golden Hour*,
https://doi.org/10.1007/978-3-030-26443-7_27

27.2 Injury Mechanisms

Injuries to the small intestine can occur in either blunt or penetrating abdominal trauma, It is the most common organ to be injured in penetrating trauma and is injured in about 5–16% of blunt abdominal trauma [1–3].

While surgical intervention in penetrating abdominal trauma is mostly immediate when indicated [4], there is a tendency toward delayed diagnosis and treatment in blunt trauma which increases the morbidity and mortality of such injuries [3].

In penetrating small bowel trauma, all three parts of the small intestine could be affected equally; it is also assumed that the number of holes within the loops of small intestine should be even in cases of gunshot wound (GSW), with the exception of tangential wounds [3].

In blunt trauma, certain injury mechanisms are associated with higher incidence of associated small intestine injuries, such as shear forces and compression between the abdominal wall and the spine that can lead to rupture of the small intestine which can also occur in blast injuries due to the sudden increase in intraluminal pressure [1].

The presence of certain signs on physical examination should alert the healthcare provider to the higher possibility of small intestine injury; these include the seat belt sign (echymosis of the abdominal wall at the area of contact with the seat belt indicating that the intestines might have been crushed between the seat belt and the spine) and the presence of chance fracture (transverse fracture of the vertebral bodies of the lower thoracic or lumbar spine [7–9].

Blunt trauma, small bowel injuries occur in about 5–16% of blunt abdominal trauma, with certain mechanisms carrying a higher risk of injuries than others, namely crushed injuries, where the abdomen is being crushed against a hard surface; this subjects the small intestine to compression against the spine leading to sudden increase in the intraluminal pressure and rupture [1].

The presence of a seatbelt sign indicates increased risk of associated small intestine injury, due to the transient occlusion of the small intestine and the sudden increase in the intraluminal pressure leading to rupture of the small intestine in certain cases [5, 6].

The presence of chance fractures (transverse fracture of the vertebral bodies of the lower thoracic or lumbar spine) might also indicate the presence of small intestine injuries [7–9].

In penetrating abdominal trauma, almost all patients subject to GSW injury to the abdomen end up with an exploratory laparotomy, wherein small bowel injury is identified and treated accordingly. It is of paramount importance to examine the entirety of the intestine including all three parts (duodenum, jejunum, and ileum) as all are equally vulnerable to injury in penetrating trauma. Also, the number of holes in the intestine should be even, with the exception of tangential injuries.

In the case of stab wounds to the abdomen, the majority of cases do not require an immediate exploratory laparotomy; those patients should be examined serially for the first 12–24 hours looking for change in symptoms or development of signs of peritonitis, preferably by the same person in order to recognize changes in abdominal examination, as patients with small bowel injury become almost always symptomatic in 6–12 hours [13]. This approach has a specificity reaching up to

100% in conscious patients [11]. Should the patient develop peritonitis, exploratory laparotomy is indicated and should not be postponed [12].

In blunt abdominal trauma, the diagnosis is more challenging due to the presence of other confounding injuries. Careful evaluation, including history to include the mechanism of injury and physical examination looking for signs of peritonitis or those associated with increased risk of small bowel injury, is made.

FAST examination, although helpful in detecting intraperitoneal bleeding in the hemodynamically unstable patients, is of limited value in detecting hollow viscus injury, especially at the early stage following the trauma.

27.3   CT Scan

In patients who are hemodynamically stable, CT scan with IV contrasts and with or without oral contrast has been frequently used as a complementary method to the anamnesis and careful physical examination in determining the need for surgical treatment.

In blunt abdominal trauma, CT scan has a sensitivity of 92%, a specificity of 94% [14], and an accuracy of 82% in detecting small intestine injuries [10]. CT scan findings of small intestine injuries most frequently found are discontinuity, edema, and alterations in the intestine wall [12]. Other findings such as extraluminal air or contrast are highly specific but have a low sensitivity. Another important and frequent finding is the presence of free fluid without obvious solid organ injury.

CT scan is less used in penetrating trauma [10]. It is important to emphasize that in penetrating trauma, the presence of an isolated finding of extraluminal air bubbles does not mean a hollow viscus injury, as it might be the result of the trajectory of the GSW or the stab wound. The most accurate finding of injury on CT scan in such cases is the extension of the trajectory of the wound itself to the bowel wall (Figs. 27.1 and 27.2) [14].

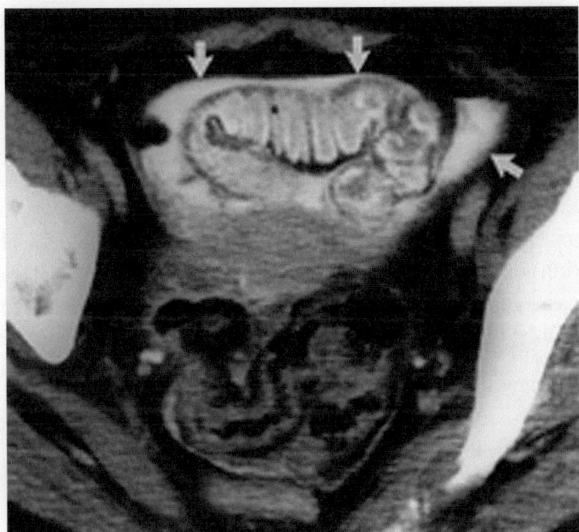

Fig. 27.1 CT showing duodenum perforation. A great contrast quantity leaking around the loop can be observed

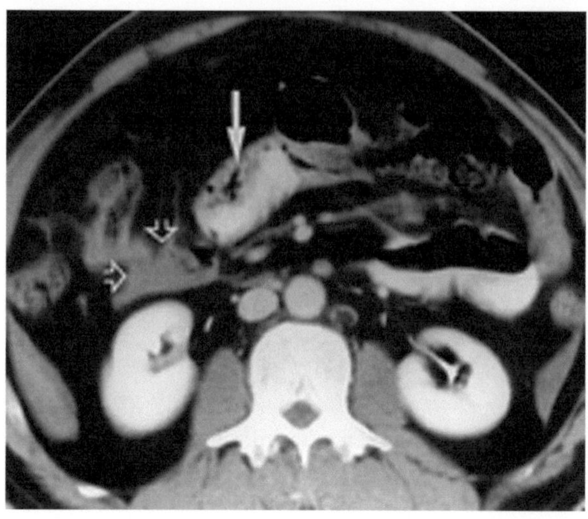

Fig. 27.2 CT showing edema of the loop wall and perforation, with pneumoperitoneum and free fluid

27.4 Treatment

The treatment of traumatic small bowel injuries is surgical, and depends on the extent of the injury. Partial thickness injuries, with an intact mucosa and no evidence of perforation, can be managed with seromuscular sutures to close the defect and re-enforce the injured area. This could be done either in an interrupted or in a continuous fashion [15].

Full-thickness injuries are dependent on the extent of the circumference involved; injuries involving less than 50% of the circumference can be managed by debridement of the edges and primary closure. If there are two contiguous holes, they should be preferably converted into one [15]. If the injury involves more than 50% of the circumference, primary closure in a transverse fashion, to avoid future strictures, is an option. This is especially valid in the jejunum as it has a wider lumen [12], whereas resection and anastomosis are preferable in cases where the distal ileum is injured as it has a smaller diameter and thus a higher risk of stenosis following primary repair [15]. The anastomosis is done either manually or using staplers depending on the availability and the preference of the surgeon. This is usually done as a side-to-side (functional end-to-end) anastomosis or as an end-to-end anastomosis in one or two layers [12, 15]. Regardless of the method used, the risk of anastomotic leak should be less than 2% (1–2%) [15]. The risk of intestinal obstruction varies and has been reported as anywhere between 0.3% and 26.9% [16]. In cases of delayed diagnosis beyond 6 hours, the presence of diffuse peritonitis along with systemic signs of sepsis is common, and in such cases, multiple laparotomies with washouts and/or diversion with an ostomy might be indicated [17–21].

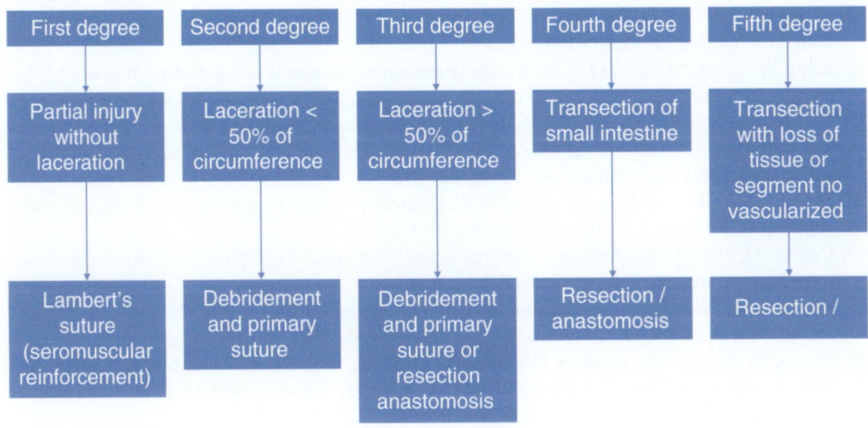

References

1. Fraga GP, Silva FHBS, Almeida NA, Curi JCM, Mantovani M. Blunt abdominal trauma with small bowel injury: are isolated lesions riskier than associated lesions? Acta Cirúrgica Brasileira. 2008;23(2):192–7.
2. Mukhopadhyay M. Intestinal injury from blunt abdominal trauma: a study of 47 cases. Oman Med J. 2009;24(4):256–9.
3. Cripps NPJ, Cooper GJ. Intestinal injury mechanisms after blunt abdominal impact. Ann R Coll Surg Engl. 2007;79:115–20.
4. Biffl W, Leppaniemi A. Management guidelines for penetrating abdominal trauma. World J Surg. 2014; https://doi.org/10.1007/s00268-014-2793-7.
5. Dowd VO, Kiernan C, Lowery A, Khan W, Barry K. Seatbelt injury causing small bowel devascularisation: case series and review of the literature. Emerg Med Int. 2011; Article ID 675341; https://doi.org/10.1155/2011/675341.
6. Vailas MG, Morir D, Orfanos S, Vergadis C, Papalambros A. Seatbelt sign in a case of blunt abdominal trauma; what lies beneath it ? BMC Surg. 2015;15:121.
7. Green DA, Green NE, Spengler DM, Devito DP. Flexion-distraction injuries to the lumbar spine associated with abdominal injuries. J Spinal Disord. 1991;4:312–8.
8. Neugebauer H, Wallenboeck E, Hungerford M. Seventy cases of injuries of the small intestine caused by blunt abdominal trauma: a retrospective study from 1970 to 1994. J Trauma. 1999;46:116–21.
9. Ritchie WP, Ersek RA, Bunch WL, Simmons RL. Combined visceral and vertebral injuries from lap type seat belts. Surg Gynecol Obstet. 1970;131:431–5.
10. Jansen JO, Yule SR, Loudon MA. Investigation of blunt abdominal trauma. BMJ. 2008;336:938–42.
11. Mefire AC, Weledji PE, Verla VS, Lidwine NM. Diagnostic and therapeutic challenges of isolated small bowel perforations after blunt abdominal injury in low income settings: analysis of twenty three new cases. Inj Int J Care Inj. 2014;45:141–5.
12. Barnett RE, Love KM, Sepulvueda EA, Cheadle WG. Small bowel trauma: current approach to diagnosis and management. Am Surg. 2014;80:1183–91.
13. Feliciano DV. Abdominal trauma revisited. Am Surg. 2017;82:1993–202.
14. Filho ELM, Mazepa MM, Guetter CR, Pimentel SK. The role of computerized tomography in penetrating abdominal trauma. Rev Col Bras Cir. 2018;45(1):e1348.

15. Weinberg JA, Croce MA. Penetrating injuries to the stomach, duodenum, and small bowel. Curr Trauma Rep. 2015;1:107–12.
16. Kang WS, Park YC, Jo YG, Kim JC. Early postoperative small bowel obstruction after laparotomy for trauma: incidence and risk factors. Ann Surg Treat Res. 2018;94(2):94–101.
17. Mefire AC, Weledji PE, Verla VS, Lidwine NM. Diagnostic and therapeutic challenges of isolated small bowel perforations after blunt abdominal injury in low income settings: analysis of twenty three new cases/ Injury. Int J Care Inj. 2014;45:141–5.
18. Morre KL, Dalleyll AF, Baltimore AMRA. Clinically oriented anatomy, vol. 7. Philadelphia: Lippincott Williams & Wilkins; 2014: chapter 2.
19. Collins JT, Bhimji SS. Anatomy, abdomen, small intestine. StatPearls 2018. Available from: https://www.ncbi.nlm.nih.gov/books/NBK459366/.
20. Whitehouse JS, Weigelt JA. Diagnostic peritoneal lavage: a review of indications, technique, and interpretation. Scand J Trauma Resusc Emerg Med. 2009;17:13.
21. Kumar S, Bnasal VK, Muduly DK, Sharma P, Misra MC, Chumber S, Singh S, Bhardwaj DN. Accuracy of focused assessment with sonography for trauma (FAST) in blunt trauma abdomen—a prospective study. Indian J Surg. 2015;77(2):393–7.

Pancreatic and Duodenal Trauma

Leonardo Yoshida Osaku, Imad Izat El Tawil,
Nelson Fernandes de Souza Jr, Mariana F. Jucá Moscardi,
and Antonio Marttos

28.1 Introduction

Traumatic injuries to the pancreas and duodenum are rare, corresponding to approximately 5–10% of abdominal trauma. Most of them are related to multiple injuries due to their close contact with pancreas, vascular structures, and other organs. Both clinical and complementary diagnoses are unspecific and late. This explains the high mortality rates, which can reach up to 30% in complex lesions.

Therefore, the following algorithm clearly explain the main conducts in front of this kind of patient.

L. Y. Osaku
Iwan Collaço Trauma Research Group, Department of Surgery, Hospital do Trabalhador Trauma Center, Federal University of Parana, Curitiba, Brazil

I. I. El Tawil · N. F. de Souza Jr
Department of Surgery, Hospital do Trabalhador Trauma Center, Federal University of Parana, Curitiba, Brazil

M. F. Jucá Moscardi (✉)
Telemedicine and Trauma Research, University of Miami, Ryder Trauma Center, Miami, FL, USA

A. Marttos
William Lehman Injury Research Center, Division of Trauma & Surgical Critical Care, Dewitt Daughtry Department of Surgery, Leonard M. Miller School of Medicine Miami, University of Miami, Miami, FL, USA

© Springer Nature Switzerland AG 2020
A. Nasr et al. (eds.), *The Trauma Golden Hour*,
https://doi.org/10.1007/978-3-030-26443-7_28

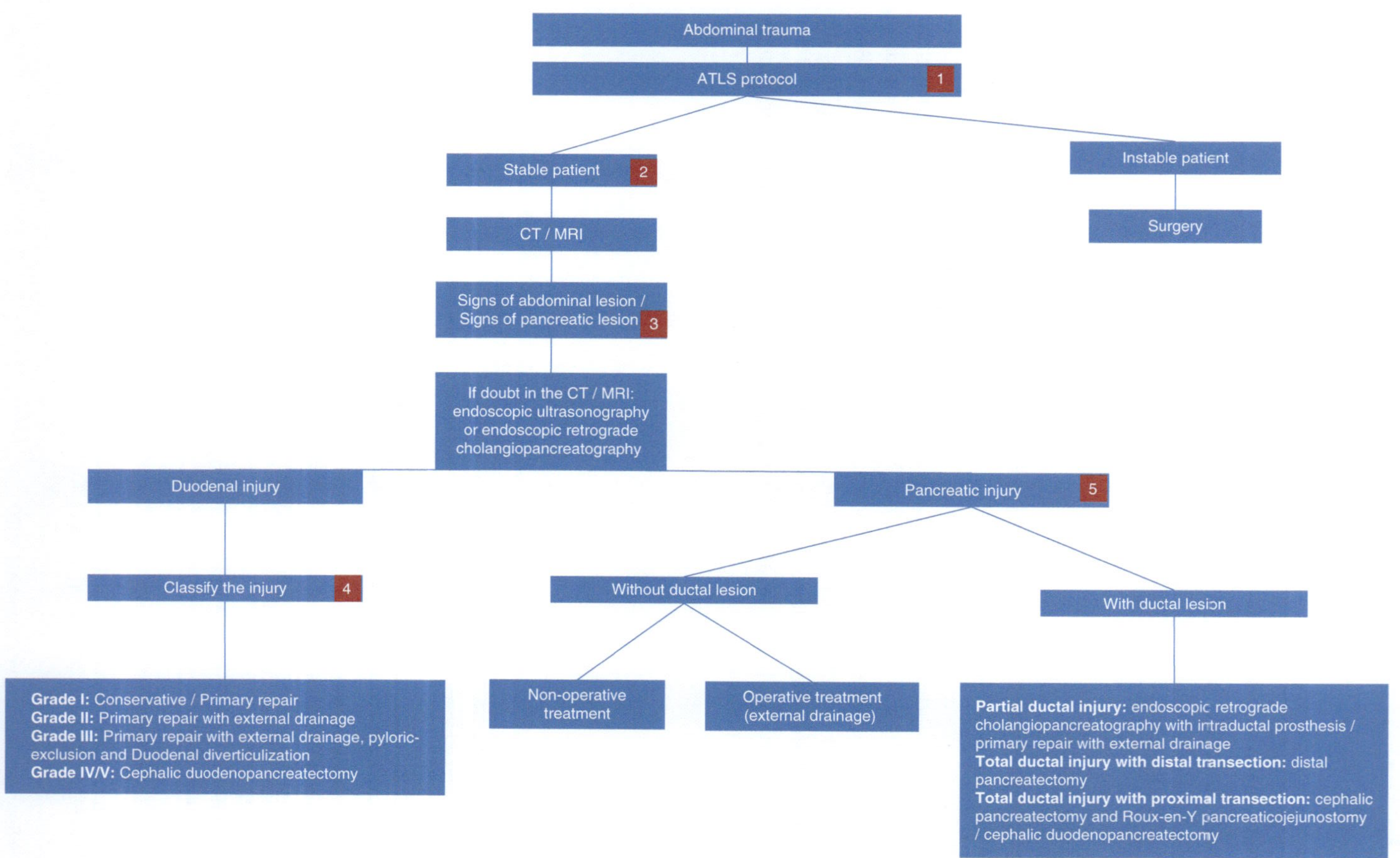

Abdominal trauma
ATLS protocol 1
Stable patient 2
Instable patient
Surgery
CT / MRI
Signs of abdominal lesion / Signs of pancreatic lesion 3
If doubt in the CT / MRI: endoscopic ultrasonography or endoscopic retrograde cholangiopancreatography
Duodenal injury
Pancreatic injury 5
Classify the injury 4
Without ductal lesion
With ductal lesion
Non-operative treatment
Operative treatment (external drainage)
Grade I: Conservative / Primary repair
Grade II: Primary repair with external drainage
Grade III: Primary repair with external drainage, pyloric-exclusion and Duodenal diverticulization
Grade IV/V: Cephalic duodenopancreatectomy
Partial ductal injury: endoscopic retrograde cholangiopancreatography with intraductal prosthesis / primary repair with external drainage
Total ductal injury with distal transection: distal pancreatectomy
Total ductal injury with proximal transection: cephalic pancreatectomy and Roux-en-Y pancreaticojejunostomy / cephalic duodenopancreatectomy

28.2 Conclusion

(1) Every trauma victim should initially be assessed according to the protocol established by ATLS. Its conducts are mainly based on the airway control, ventilation, and hemodynamic status.

(2) Hemodynamically stable patient is the one who presents blood pressure greater than 90 mmHg and maintains it for at least one hour, not requiring new fluid replacement of vasopressor drugs.

(3) Signs of duodenal injury: pneumoperitoneum, penumoretroperitoneum, free fluid, increased space between the right kidney and duodenum. Signs of pancreatic lesion: pneumoperitoneum, air at the lower pole of the right kidney, retropsoas air, L1–L2 fracture.

(4) Duodenal injuries may be graded according to the AAST classification.

Grade	Injury	Description
I	Hematoma	Single portion of duodenum
	Laceration	Partial thickness only
II	Hematoma	Involving more than one portion
	Laceration	Disruption of <50% of circumference
III	Laceration	Disruption of 50–70% of the circumference of D2 Disruption of 50–100% of the circumference of D1, D3, and D4
IV	Laceration	Disruption of <75% of the circumference of D2 involving the ampulla of distal common duct
V	Laceration	Massive disruption of the duodenopancreatic complex
	Vascular	Devascularization of the duodenum

(5) Pancreatic injuries may be graded according to the AAST classification.

Pancreatic injuries		
Grade	Type of injury	Description of injury
I	Hematoma	Minor contusion without duct injury
	Laceration	Superficial laceration without duct injury
II	Hematoma	Major contusion without duct injury or tissue loss
	Laceration	Major laceration without duct injury or tissue loss
III	Laceration	Distal transection or parenchymal injury with duct injury
IV	Laceration	Proximal transection or parenchymal injury involving ampulla
V	Laceration	Massive disruption of pancreatic head

Bibliography

1. Asensio JA, Petrone P, Roldán R, Pak-art R, Salim A. Pancreatic and duodenal injuries. Complex and lethal. Scand J Surg. 2002;91:81–6.
2. Ker-Kan T, Chan DX, Vijayan A, Ming-Terk C. Management of pancreatic injuries after blunt abdominal trauma. Experience at a single institution. J Pancreas (Online). 2009;10(6):657–63.
3. Gupta V, Wig JD, Garg H. Trauma pancreaticoduodenectomy for complex pancreaticoduodenal injury. Delayed reconstruction. J Pancreas (Online). 2008;9(5):618–23.
4. Ahmad I, Branicki FJ, Ramadhan K, El-Ashaal Y, Abu-Zidan FM. Pancreatic injuries in the United Arab Emirates. Scand J Surg. 2008;97:243–7.
5. Moncoure M, Goins WA. Challenges in the management of Pancreatic and Duodenal Injuries. J Natl Med Assoc. 1993;85(10):767–72.
6. Feliciano D, Mattox K, Moore E. Trauma. New York: McGraw-Hill Professional; 2007.

Colon Injuries

29

Rafaela de Araújo Molteni, Waleyd Ahmad Omar,
Rached Hajar Traya, Mariana F. Jucá Moscardi,
Yukihiro Kanda, and Rishi Rattan

29.1 Introduction

The majority of colon injuries are caused by penetrating trauma. In penetrating trauma, the colon is the second most injured organ, next to the small intestine. In abdominal gunshot wounds, the colon is involved in approximately 27% of cases undergoing laparotomy. In blunt abdominal trauma, less than 5% of patients suffer colon injuries. The repair of colon injuries remains one of the most controversial subjects among trauma surgeons. Of note, for the purposes of surgical management of injury, the intraperitoneal rectum should be treated similarly to the colon.

Historically, the management of colon injuries was developed in military settings and later extrapolated to the civilian population. During World War I, studies regarding the best way to repair colon injuries initially reported that while minor injuries could be primarily repaired, resection and primary anastomosis resulted in poor outcomes. Colostomy was seen as safest. During World War II, despite better technology, antibiotics, and infrastructure, colostomy was still widely performed. However, in the proceeding decades, largely as a result of the Korean and Vietnam Wars, the exteriorized repair became popular. A primary resection and anastomosis

R. de Araújo Molteni · W. A. Omar · R. H. Traya
Department of Surgery, Hospital do Trabalhador Trauma Center,
Federal University of Parana, Curitiba, Brazil

M. F. Jucá Moscardi (✉)
Telemedicine and Trauma Research, University of Miami, Ryder Trauma Center,
Miami, FL, USA

Y. Kanda
Ryder Trauma Center – Jackson Health System, Miller School of Medicine, University of
Miami, Miami, FL, USA

R. Rattan
Division of Trauma Surgery & Critical Care, DeWitt Daughtry Family Department of
Surgery, Miller School of Medicine, University of Miami, Miami, FL, USA

© Springer Nature Switzerland AG 2020
A. Nasr et al. (eds.), *The Trauma Golden Hour*,
https://doi.org/10.1007/978-3-030-26443-7_29

were performed and exteriorized through the skin similar to a colostomy. If there was no obvious anastomotic leak, the exteriorized part was taken down and returned to the peritoneal cavity after a couple of weeks. However, this repair also had high complication rates. The finding that peritoneal contamination due to colon injury does not in and of itself necessitate colostomy in the modern era advanced alternative treatment options.

There are three treatment options for colon injuries: primary repair, resection and anastomosis, and resection and fecal diversion. The treatment of colon injuries is based on its classification according the American Association for the Surgery of Trauma (AAST), Colon Injury Scale (CIS), published by Cayten et al., and depends on the patients' conditions and risk factors.

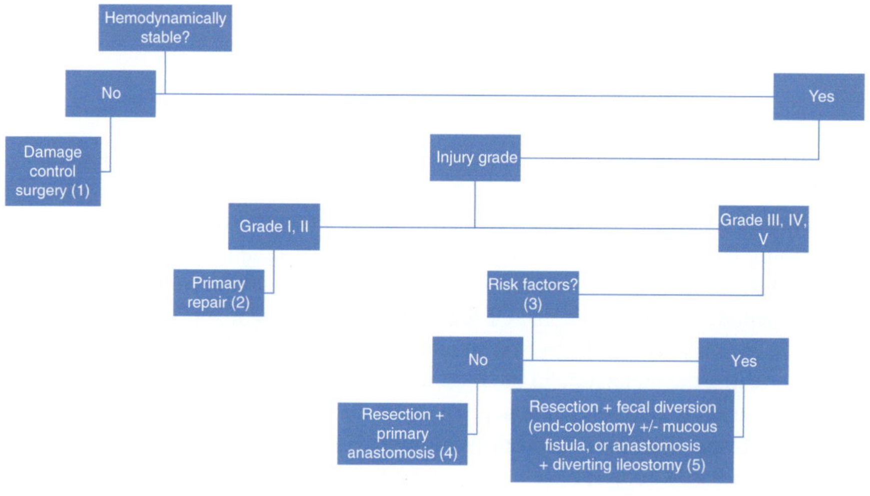

29.2 Conclusion

(1) In damage control surgeries, the repair of colon injury is performed by using cardiac tapes or staplers involving proximal and distal colon. Second-look surgery is performed when the patient has been adequately resuscitated and acidosis, coagulopathy, and hypothermia reversed, usually 12–48 hours after initial laparotomy. If a patient is physiologically stable, definitive treatment can be performed.

(2) Primary repair can be performed using absorbable or permanent suture in a single- or double-layer technique according to local practice and surgeon preference.

(3) Risk factors include hemodynamic instability, transfusion of more than 4 units of blood within the first 24 hours, significant associated injuries, and diffuse fecal contamination.

(4) In case of injuries close to the middle colic artery, one must consider the need to perform extended hemicolectomy based on remaining blood supply. The

method of anastomosis (handsewn or stapled anastomosis) does not affect the incidence of abdominal complications.

(5) Resection and anastomosis with diverting ileostomy may have acceptable morbidity and mortality with relatively less morbidity and early reversal of stoma when compared to end-colostomy but consideration of resources, including ability to percutaneously drain any possible resulting intraabdominal infections and follow-up, must be taken into consideration.

Bibliography

1. Demetriades D, Benjamin E, Inaba K. Colon and rectal trauma. In: Moore EE, Feliciano DV, Mattox KL, editors. Trauma. 8th ed. New York: McGraw-Hill; 2017. p. 639–49.
2. Eastern Association for the Surgery of Trauma. EAST practice management guidelines, colon injuries, penetrating. 1998. https://www.east.org/education/practice-management-guidelines/colon-injuries-penetrating.
3. Demetriades D, Murray JA, Chan L, et al. Penetrating colon injuries requiring resection: diversion or primary anastomosis? An AAST prospective multicenter study. J Trauma. 2001;50:765–75.
4. Demetriades D, Murray JA, Chan LS, et al. Handsewn versus stapled anastomosis in penetrating colon injuries requiring resection: a multicenter study. J Trauma. 2002;52:117–21.
5. Gala T, Tufail R, Murtaza G, et al. Role of protective stoma in destructive colon injuries in gunshot victims and predictors of post-operative morbidity in a developing country. Ann Surg Perioper Care. 2017;2:1032.

Rectum and Perineum Injuries

30

Rafaela de Araújo Molteni, Fábio Henrique de Carvalho, Janaina de Oliveira Poy, April Anne Grant, and Rishi Rattan

30.1 Introduction

Rectal injuries are less frequent than colon injuries and management has dramatically evolved over the last half century. A recent review done by the American Association for the Surgery of Trauma (AAST) was published in 2018, and describes well the evolution of management.

It is now accepted that intraperitoneal rectal injuries should be treated as abdominal colonic injuries. Therefore, this is discussed in the chapter on colonic injuries.

We will focus on extraperitoneal rectal injuries. The extraperitoneal rectum is surrounded and protected by the bony pelvis. It lies in close proximity to many of the structures of the genitourinary tract, which can make repair difficult. Associated lesions are common and should always be searched for based on the trauma mechanism. Historically, rectal injuries were managed with the "4 D's": *diversion*, presacral *drainage*, *direct repair*, and *distal washout* [1]. However, this is evolving and lack of benefit, and even harm, has been documented with routine pre-sacral drainage and distal washout; therefore, routine drainage and distal rectal washout are no longer recommended [2, 3]. Diversion has proven to be the most beneficial approach

R. de Araújo Molteni · F. H. de Carvalho
Department of Surgery, Hospital do Trabalhador Trauma Center,
Federal University of Parana, Curitiba, Brazil

J. de Oliveira Poy
Faculdade de Ciências Médicas de Santos, Santos, São Paulo, Brazil

A. A. Grant
Ryder Trauma Center – Jackson Health System, Miller School of Medicine, University of Miami, Miami, FL, USA

R. Rattan (✉)
Division of Trauma Surgery & Critical Care, DeWitt Daughtry Family Department of Surgery, Miller School of Medicine, University of Miami, Miami, FL, USA
e-mail: rrattan@miami.edu

© Springer Nature Switzerland AG 2020
A. Nasr et al. (eds.), *The Trauma Golden Hour*,
https://doi.org/10.1007/978-3-030-26443-7_30

in the management of these lesions. Direct repair has not been shown to be beneficial, but no harm has been demonstrated either, so additional study is warranted to see which patient population would most benefit from direct repair [3].

Complex perineal lesions continue to represent a challenge and their treatment requires multidisciplinary support. These lesions frequently result from high-energy trauma and have high morbidity and mortality rates. Damage control surgery for hemorrhage and contamination is the first priority with staged procedures for reconstruction after patient stabilization.

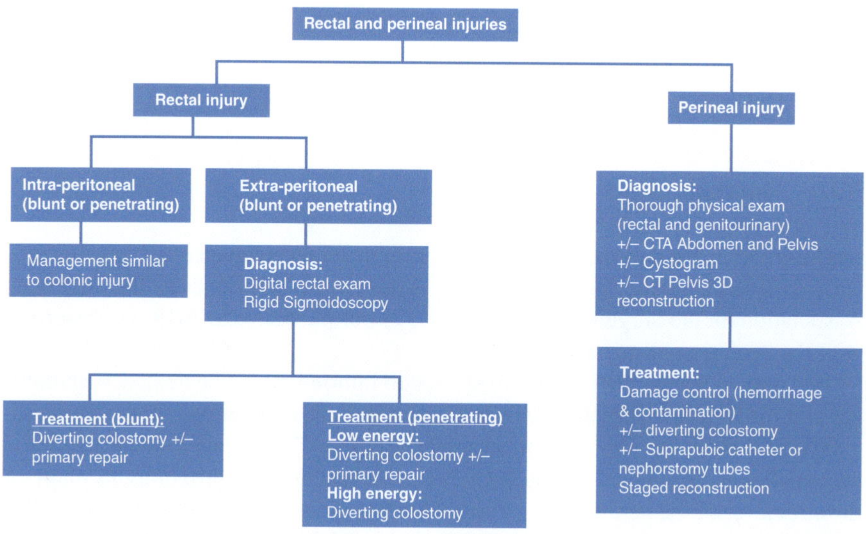

30.2　Conclusion

(1) The diagnosis of rectal injury can be difficult and requires a high index of suspicion particularly for blunt mechanism. More important than the distinction of mechanism (blunt or penetrating) is the location of the rectal injury. Intraperitoneal injuries are treated as colonic injuries regardless of mechanism. Extraperitoneal injuries require additional thought and different management.

(2) The presence of blood during the digital rectal exam is an important sign. Rigid sigmoidoscopy, followed by CT abdomen and pelvis were the most common diagnostic modalities utilized across a recent multicenter study [3]. Diagnostic choice depends on the stability of the victim and resource availability.

(3) If an extraperitoneal injury is identified, the standard of care is to perform a diverting colostomy [3] regardless of mechanism (blunt or penetrating). While some reports of primary repair without diverting colostomy can be found in the literature, evidence does not currently support this shift in the management of these injuries [4, 5]. Extensive dissection to search a lesion is discouraged due to enlarging of the dead space, increasing the risk of bleeding and causing nerve damage. As stated above, neither pre-sacral drainage nor the irrigation of the

distal rectal stump is recommended [2, 3]. Associated injuries are frequent and should be treated accordingly with appropriate specialty consultation.

(4) Simple perineal injuries to soft tissue associated with low-energy mechanism can be repaired primarily. Complex perineal trauma comprises injuries that often include injuries to the soft tissue, genitourinary tract, rectum, vascular system, and bony pelvis. A high index of suspicion for injury and rapid diagnosis of injury to any of these structures is paramount. Diagnostic modalities utilized will depend upon the index of suspicion of injury and thorough evaluations of the rectum, genitourinary tract, vascular system, and bony pelvis. In a stable patient, the most common initial imaging at a large trauma center is a CT Angio of the abdomen and pelvis followed by a CT cystogram. Appropriate consults are placed, as injuries are identified and may include orthopedic surgery for pelvic fractures, interventional radiology if extravasation from pelvic fractures is identified, urology, gynecology, colorectal surgery, and eventually, plastic surgery.

(5) The ability to perform definitive repair depends on several factors including patient stability, degree of contamination, and availability of specialists. Typically, complex perineal injuries require multiple staged procedures. In an unstable patient, damage control surgery is performed with control of hemorrhage and contamination being the chief goals. Procedures that are needed may include ligation of bleeding vessels, debridement of devitalized tissue, possible revascularization, and diversion of the GI and GU tract as needed (ostomy and/or suprapubic urinary catheter or nephrostomy tubes). Serial washouts of the wound are often necessary and staged reconstruction occurs over the next several days to weeks as the patient stabilizes. Treatment is most often multidisciplinary and may require the skills of urology, colorectal surgery, gynecology, vascular surgery, or plastic surgery for reconstruction. The trauma surgeon's role is immediate damage control and overseeing the complex repair of these severe multi-trauma injuries.

References

1. Lavenson GS, Cohen A. Management of rectal injuries. Am J Surg. 1971;122:226–30.
2. Bosarge PL, Como JJ, Fox N, Falck-Ytter Y, Hunt ER, Dorion HA, Patel NJ, Rushing A, Raff LA, McDonald AA, Robinson BRH, McGwin G, Bonzalez RP. Management of penetrating extraperitoneal rectal injuries: an Eastern Association for the Surgery of Trauma practice management guidelines. J Trauma. 2016;80:546–51.
3. Brown CVR, Teixeira PG, Furay E, Sharpe JP, Musonza T, Holcomb J, Bui E, Bruns B, Hopper A, Truitt MS, Burlew CC, Schellenberg M, Sava J, VanHorn J, Eastridge B, Cross A, Vasak R, Vercruysse G, Curtis EE, Haan J, Coimbra R, Bohan P, Gale S, Bendix PG. Contemporary management of rectal injuries at Level I trauma centers: the results of the American Association for the Surgery of Trauma multi-institutional study. J Trauma. 2018;84(2):225–33.
4. Gonzalez RP, Phelan H III, Hassan M, Ellis CN, Rodning CV. Is fecal diversion necessary for nondestructive penetrating extraperitoneal rectal lesions? J Trauma. 2006;61:815–9.
5. Levine JH, Long WE, Pruitt C, Mazuski JE, Shapiro MJ, Durham RM. Management of selected rectal injuries by primary repair. Am J Surg. 1996;172:575–9.

Abdominal Vascular Lesions 31

Ana Gabriela Clemente da Silva, Paola Zarur Varella,
Alan Cesar Diorio, Márcio Luciano Canevari Filho,
Cristiano Silva Pinto, April Anne Grant,
and Gerrard Daniel Pust

31.1 Introduction

This chapter aims to standardize the care of patients treated at the Worker's Hospital with suspected or confirmed abdominal vascular injury. The protocol will cover the lesions of the following intraabdominal vessels: aorta, inferior vena cava, portal vein, and iliac vessels. This standardization is important because, even in a trauma center, the care of patients with abdominal vascular trauma is infrequent, since most die before reaching the hospital [1].

The penetrating trauma corresponds to the great majority of lesions, which may present as thrombosis, contained hematomas, active bleeding, pseudoaneurysms, or arteriovenous fistulas. Regardless of the mechanism of trauma, the presence of associated lesions is extremely frequent [2].

When should we suspect an abdominal vascular injury? Penetrating abdominal trauma associated with severe hypovolemic shock, presence of active external bleeding, pulsatile hematoma, murmur or thrill, suspicious trajectory,

A. G. C. da Silva · M. L. C. Filho
Iwan Collaço Trauma Research Group, Department of Surgery, Hospital do Trabalhador
Trauma Center, Federal University of Parana, Curitiba, Brazil

P. Z. Varella · A. C. Diorio · C. S. Pinto
Department of Surgery, Hospital do Trabalhador Trauma Center,
Federal University of Parana, Curitiba, Brazil

A. A. Grant
Ryder Trauma Center – Jackson Health System, Miller School of Medicine, University of
Miami, Miami, FL, USA

G. D. Pust (✉)
Division of Trauma Surgery & Critical Care, DeWitt Daughtry Family Department of
Surgery, Miller School of Medicine, University of Miami, Miami, FL, USA
e-mail: gpust@med.miami.edu

© Springer Nature Switzerland AG 2020
A. Nasr et al. (eds.), *The Trauma Golden Hour*,
https://doi.org/10.1007/978-3-030-26443-7_31

location of a suspected projectile, reduction or absence of pulse distal to injury, signs of ischemia, or venous insufficiency distal to injury. Before the suspicion of an abdominal vascular injury, one should immediately contact the vascular surgeon on call.

As in any trauma patient, after initial care according to the ATLS, he/she should be classified for hemodynamic stability. In hemodynamically stable patients, we can use complementary tests to plan the best treatment. Among the main exams, we can mention simple Rx, Doppler ultrasonography, computed tomography, and arteriography, the latter being considered a "gold standard" [3–6]. In contrast, unstable patients with suspected abdominal vascular injury should be taken to the surgical center immediately [6].

The use of antibiotics is recommended at the anesthetic induction. The antisepsis should be performed throughout the trunk, by the possibility of needing a thoracic drainage or thoracotomy, and in the proximal part of the thighs if a saphenous vein is needed to repair a vascular lesion. The laparotomy should be wide. In the presence of a retroperitoneal hematoma, proximal and distal control should be performed before the direct approach to the hematoma. In cases of hemoperitoneum, the four quadrants of the abdomen should be tamponed with compresses, which, after removal, will allow the identification of the lesion [7]. The active bleeding can be compressed with the finger itself, with gases mounted or using vascular clamp. The proximal and distal control of the vessel is then done wherever possible. Blind clamping of a bleeding vessel should be avoided because of the risk of further injury [8].

There are some basic principles that guide the repair of a vascular injury: whenever the injury is due to a firearm projectile injury, it is necessary to debride its edges before repairing. In addition, the raffia of the lesion is made with polypropylene yarn and should always follow the transverse direction of the vessel, so as to avoid its stenosis [9]. In the stable patient with associated hollow viscus lesion, the control of the bleeding and the repair of the viscus are performed, followed by washing the cavity, changing the gloves and, finally, the vascular repair [10].

Vascular damage control surgery is indicated when vascular injury is complex and the patient remains hemodynamically unstable. Damage control can be accomplished through shunts, bandages, or tamponades. A shunt can be made by interposing a plastic tube, a nasogastric tube, or a chest tube. This is fixed in the proximal and distal segments of the vessel, which will allow the flow to remain provisionally until the definitive repair of the lesion is performed [11].

Thoracotomy for clamping the aorta in order to avoid abdominal exsanguination can be performed [12–14].

Faced with an abdominal aortic injury, we must perform the Mattox maneuver. This allows adequate exposure of the aorta from the celiac trunk to the iliac bifurcation. Whenever possible, we must make the primary repair of the lesion, provided that it does not present a risk of stenosis of the vessel. In these cases, vessel mobilization followed by end-to-end anastomosis or the use of Dacron prostheses are the best options [6, 14, 15]. Saphenous vein grafts, bovine pericardium, or PTFE grafts may also be used for repair of a partial injury [14]. Extra-anatomical shunts should be reserved for exceptional situations, among them the presence of massive abdominal contamination [16].

The repair of a lesion in the inferior vena cava should take into account the height of the lesion. The Cattell maneuver allows exposure of the entire infrahepatic vena cava. Whenever possible, primary suture should be employed, especially in the adrenal segment. The inferior vena cava tolerates a reduction of up to 75% of its lumen [15]. In smaller diameters, it is prudent to use grafts, which may be saphenous from the patient as well as synthetic materials such as PTFE and Dacron [17, 18]. In extensive lesions of the infrarenal vena cava, ligature of the vessel is a viable resource due to the lumbar vein's capacity of developing sufficient collateral circulation to supply the venous return of the lower limbs and pelvis. In cases of retro-hepatic vena cava injury, compressed tamponade followed by a *second look* for definitive repair of the lesion is the option associated with a lower mortality rate [19].

Injuries to the portal vein are technically difficult to repair due to massive bleeding and the presence of lesions associated with its anatomical position. Patients suspected of having a portal vein lesion should undergo a Kocher maneuver. The minor lesions can be submitted to primary suture. In case of larger lesions, usually associated with hemodynamic instability, the ligature should be considered. In this situation, a *second look* should be performed for the possibility of ischemia or intestinal infarction [20].

For the correction of lesions of the iliac arteries, besides the primary suture and the use of synthetic grafts, there are possibilities of arterial transpositions and contralateral reimplantations, as well as bridges and interpositions using the saphenous vein of the patient. In extreme situations, the placement of a shunt or even the ligature should be considered [14, 21, 22].

In very specific situations, endovascular treatment may be a great option for several abdominal vascular injuries.

Algorithms

Abdominal Trauma with Vascular lesion suspected
Call Vascular Surgeon
Emergency room
Unstable
Surgery
Stable
Angiotomography
Results
Vascular lesion
Doubt
Arteriography
Normal
Normal
Exclude Vascular Lesion

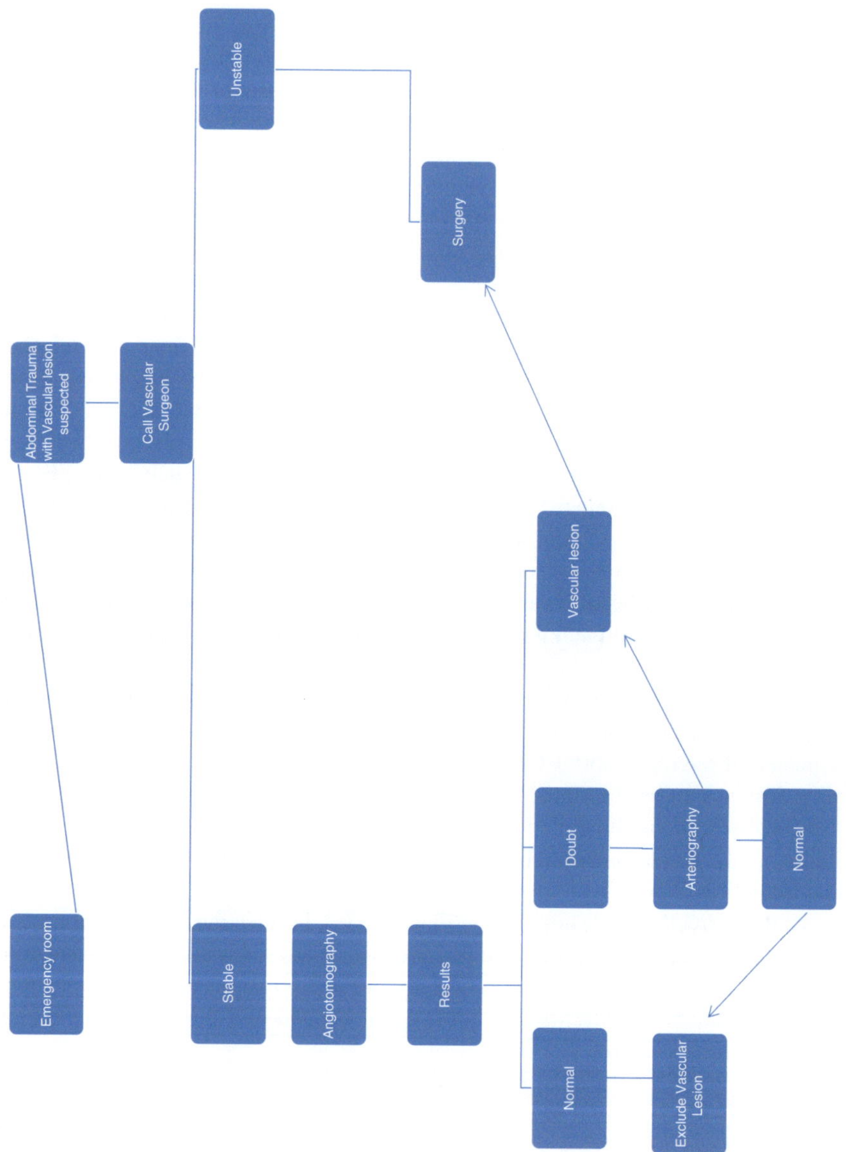

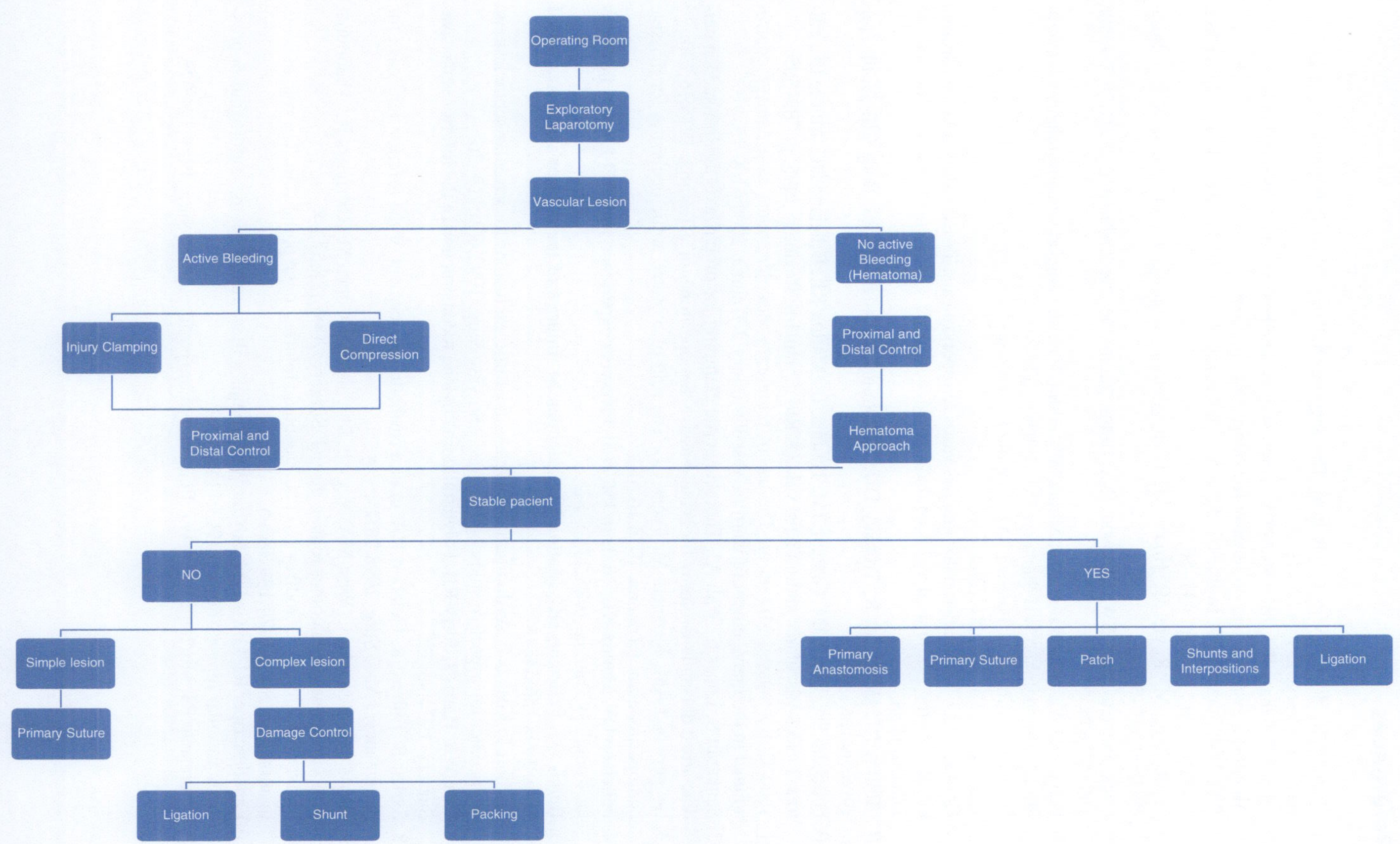

Operating Room
Exploratory Laparotomy
Vascular Lesion
Active Bleeding
No active Bleeding (Hematoma)
Injury Clamping
Direct Compression
Proximal and Distal Control
Proximal and Distal Control
Hematoma Approach
Stable pacient
NO
YES
Simple lesion
Complex lesion
Primary Suture
Damage Control
Ligation
Shunt
Packing
Primary Anastomosis
Primary Suture
Patch
Shunts and Interpositions
Ligation

References

1. Coimbra R, Hoyt D, Winchell R, et al. The ongoing challenge of retroperitoneal vascular injuries. Am J Surg. 1996;172:541–5.
2. Silva LF, Sahagoff J, Mendes WDS. Trauma vascular. In: Rossi M, editor. Trauma de Aorta Abdominal, vol. 38. Rio de Janeiro: Revinter; 2006. p. 358p.
3. Rich NM, Spencer FC. Injuries of the abdominal aorta. In: Vascular trauma. Philadelphia: WB Saunders Co.; 1978. p. 441–56.
4. Frydenberg M, Royle JP, Hoare M. Blunt abdominal aortic trauma. Aust N Z J Surg. 1990;60:347–50.
5. Lock JS, Huffman SW, Johnson RC. Blunt trauma to the abdominal aorta. J Trauma. 1987;27:674–7.
6. Perry MO. Vascular trauma. In: Moore WS, editor. Vascular surgery: a comprehensive review. 4th ed. Philadelphia: WB Saunders Co.; 1993. p. 638–40.
7. Hoyt DB, Coimbra R, Potenza BM, Rappold F. Anatomia exposures for vascular injuries. Surg Clin North Am. 2001;81:1299–330.
8. Gonzales EO. Traumatismo dos grandes vasos retroperitoneais. Tese de Mestrado em Cirurgia Geral – Setor Abdominal da Faculdade de Medicina da Universidade Federal do Rio de Janeiro. 1988.
9. Mullins RJ, Huckfeldt R, Trunkey DD. Abdominal vascular injuries. Surg Clin North Am. 1996;76(4):813–31.
10. Feliciano DV, Burch JM, Graham JM. Trauma. In: Mattox KL, Feliciano DC, Moore EE, editors. Lesões vasculares abdominais, vol. 35. Rio de Janeiro: Revinter; 2005. p. 783–805.
11. Todd E, Rasmussen MD, et al. The use of temporary vascular shunts as a damage control adjunct in the management of wartime vascular injury. J Trauma. 2006;61:8–15.
12. Sankaran S, Lucas C, Walt AJ. Thoracic aortic clamping for prophylaxis against sudden cardiac arrest during laparotomy for acute massive hemoperitoneum. J Trauma. 1975;15:290.
13. Ledgerwood AM, Kazmers M, Lucas CE. The role of thoracic aortic occlusion for massive hemoperitoneum. J Trauma. 1976;16:610.
14. Feliciano DV, Mattox KL, Graham JM, et al. Five-year experience with PTFE grafts in vascular wounds. J Trauma. 1985;25:71–82.
15. Burch JM, Feliciano DC, Mattox KL, Edelman M. Injuries of the inferior vena cava. Am J Surg. 1998;156:548–52.
16. Bacourt F, Koskas F. Axilobifemoral bypass and aortic exclusions for vascular septic lesions: multicenter retrospective study of 98 cases. Ann Vasc Surg. 1992;6(2):119–26.
17. Dale WA, Harris J, Terry RB. Polytetrafluoroethylene reconstruction of the inferior vena cava. Surgery. 1984;95:625.
18. Sarkar R, Eilber FR, Gelabert HA, et al. Prosthetic replacement of the inferior vena cava for malignancy. J Vasc Surg. 1998;28:75.
19. Hansen CJ, Bernadas C, West MA, Ney AL, Muehlsrdt S, Cohen M, Rodrigues JL. Abdominal vena cava injuries: outcomes remain dismal. Surgery. 2000;128:572–8.
20. Pachter HT, Drager S, Godfrey N, et al. Traumatic injuries to the portal vein. The role of acute ligation. Ann Surg. 1979;189:383–5.
21. Landdercasper RJ, Lewis DM, Snyder WH. Complex iliac arterial trauma: autologous or prosthetic vascular repair. Surgery. 1993;114:9.
22. Landreneau RJ, Mitchum P, Fry WJ. Iliac artery transposition. Arch Surg. 1989;124:978.

Traumatic Injuries to the Pelvic Ring

32

José Marcos Lavrador Filho, Marcelo Abagge,
Christiano Saliba Uliana, Beatriz Ortis Yazbek,
Mariana F. Jucá Moscardi, and Enrique Ginzburg

32.1 Introduction

The velocity era begun with the invention of the assembly line by Henry Ford, the development of the urban centers, and, posteriorly, the improvement of quality of life to the autovehicles, which modified the incidence of several types of traumas, making high-energy trauma one of the greatest evils of modern times.

Constituting 3% of all injuries of the skeleton, pelvis fractures present features that make their approach crucial at the emergency services. The mean incidence of 23 cases in 100,000 inhabitants in Brazil, the high cost of the hospitalized patient (approximately $65,000 dollars per patient in the United States), the bimodal pattern of presentation (young men and elderly women), and the severity of the cases are factors which demonstrate the importance of this injury.

In this context, injuries to the pelvic ring became very important. High morbidity and mortality rates are observed in 15–50% of the cases, and an association to multiple organ injurie is present in approximately 75% of the cases.

The standardization of polytraumatized patient's assessment and the evolution of the orthopedic approach are improving the prognosis of these cases. Therefore, we will present an algorithm of conducts for the polytraumatized patient with suspected pelvic ring fracture.

J. M. L. Filho · M. Abagge · C. S. Uliana
Department of Surgery, Hospital do Trabalhador Trauma Center, Federal University of Parana, Curitiba, Brazil

B. O. Yazbek
Faculdade de Ciências Médicas de Santos, Santos, São Paulo, Brazil

M. F. Jucá Moscardi (✉)
Telemedicine and Trauma Research, University of Miami, Ryder Trauma Center, Miami, FL, USA

E. Ginzburg
Division of Trauma Surgery & Critical Care, DeWitt Daughtry Family Department of Surgery, Miller School of Medicine, University of Miami, Miami, FL, USA

© Springer Nature Switzerland AG 2020
A. Nasr et al. (eds.), *The Trauma Golden Hour*,
https://doi.org/10.1007/978-3-030-26443-7_32

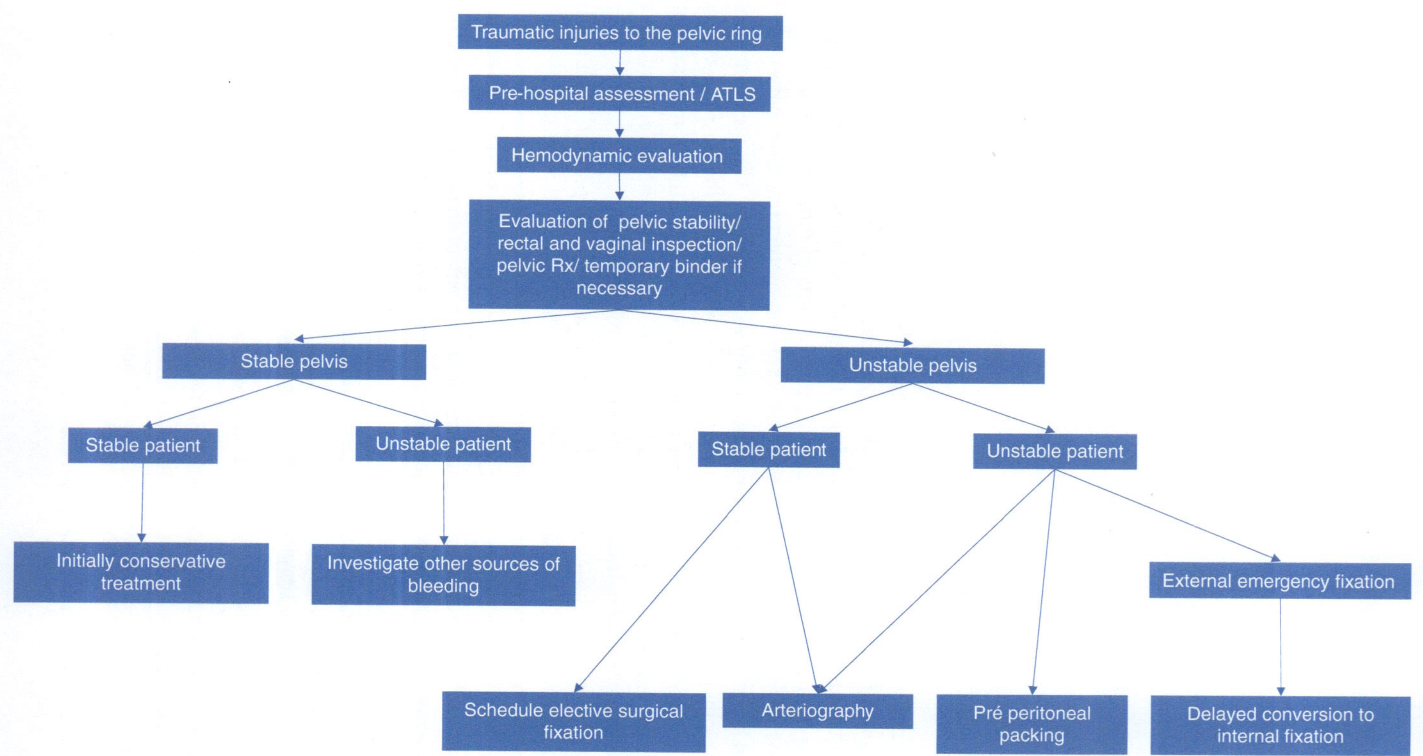

Traumatic injuries to the pelvic ring
Pre-hospital assessment / ATLS
Hemodynamic evaluation
Evaluation of pelvic stability/ rectal and vaginal inspection/ pelvic Rx/ temporary binder if necessary
Stable pelvis
Unstable pelvis
Stable patient
Unstable patient
Stable patient
Unstable patient
Initially conservative treatment
Investigate other sources of bleeding
External emergency fixation
Schedule elective surgical fixation
Arteriography
Pré peritoneal packing
Delayed conversion to internal fixation

Bibliography

1. Koval KJ, Zuckerman JD. Pelvic fractures. In: Koval KJ, Zuckerman JD, Egol KA, editors. Handbook of fractures. Philadelphia: Lippincott Williams & Wilkins (LWW); 2010. p. 327–43.
2. Gardner M, Nork S. Stabilization of unstable pelvic fractures with supraacetabular compression external fixation. J Orthop Trauma. 2007;21:269–73.
3. Kellam JF, Browner BD. Fractures of the pelvic ring. In: Browner B, Jupiter J, Levine A, Trafton P, editors. Skeletal trauma. Philadelphia: WB Saunders; 1992. p. 849–97.
4. Pohlemann T, Bosch U, Gansslen A, et al. The Hannover experience in management of pelvic fractures. Clin Orthop. 1994;1994:69–80.
5. Sevitt S. Fatal road accidents. Injuries, complications, and causes of death in 250 subjects. Br J Surg. 1968;55:481.
6. Slatis P, Karaharju EO. External fixation of the pelvic girdle with a trapezoid compression frame. Injury. 1975;7:53–6.
7. Duchesne JC, Bharmal HM, Dini AA, Islam T, Schmieg RE Jr, Simmons JD, Wahl GM, Davis JA Jr, Krause P, McSwain NE Jr. Open-book pelvic fractures with perineal open wounds: a significant morbid combination. Am Surg. 2009;75(12):1227–33.
8. Filho C, de Moraes R, et al. Fratura de pelve: um marcador de gravidade em trauma. Rev Col Bras Cir, Rio de Janeiro. 2011;38(5): pp.310-316. ISSN 0100-6991. https://doi.org/10.1590/S0100-69912011000500005.

Renal Trauma

33

Denise Magalhães Machado, Carlos Hugo Barros Cardoso,
Márcio André Sartor, Mariana F. Jucá Moscardi,
and Antonio Marttos

33.1 Introduction

Regarding genitourinary tract, the kidney is the most commonly affected organ, with injuries in 1–5% in all traumas and up to 10% in abdominal traumas [1]. Blunt trauma is more frequent with 90–95% of the kidney injuries, while penetrating trauma wounds tend to be more severe, with a higher number of associated injuries and result in a higher nephrectomy rate.

Possible renal trauma indicatives in the anamnesis and physical exam are falls, high-energy car accidents, and direct trauma to the flanks. In case of penetrating wound, information such as the size of the stab and the caliber of the gun are important. The presence of pre-existing renal abnormalities makes kidney injuries after trauma more likely. When kidney injury is suspected, an investigation with evaluation of the patient's hemodynamic status, microscopic and macroscopic

D. M. Machado
Iwan Collaço Trauma Research Group, Department of Surgery, Hospital do Trabalhador
Trauma Center, Federal University of Parana, Curitiba, Brazil

C. H. B. Cardoso · M. A. Sartor
Department of Surgery, Hospital do Trabalhador Trauma Center,
Federal University of Parana, Curitiba, Brazil

M. F. Jucá Moscardi (✉)
Telemedicine and Trauma Research, University of Miami, Ryder Trauma Center,
Miami, FL, USA

A. Marttos
William Lehman Injury Research Center, Division of Trauma & Surgical Critical Care,
Dewitt Daughtry Department of Surgery, Leonard M. Miller School of Medicine Miami,
University of Miami, Miami, FL, USA

© Springer Nature Switzerland AG 2020
A. Nasr et al. (eds.), *The Trauma Golden Hour*,
https://doi.org/10.1007/978-3-030-26443-7_33

Table 33.1 AAST Kidney Injury scale

Grade	Type of injury	Description of injury
I	Contusion Hematoma	Microscopic or gross hematuria, normal urologic studies Subcapsular, nonexpanding without parenchymal laceration
II	Hematoma Laceration	Nonexpanding perirenal hematoma confined to renal retroperitoneum <1 cm parenchymal depth of renal cortex without urinary extravasation
III	Laceration	<1 cm parenchymal depth of renal cortex without collecting system rupture or urinary extravasation
IV	Laceration Vascular	Parenchymal laceration extending through renal cortex, medula, and collecting system Main renal artery or vein injury with contained hemorrhage
V	Laceration Vascular	Completely shattered kidney Avulsion of renal hilum which devascularizes kidney

Remarks: Advance one grade for bilateral injuries up to grade III
Abbreviation: *AAST* American Association for the Surgery of Trauma
Ref: [4]

urine analysis, and, selectively, imagining exams, which will bring essential information to define the conduct, should be performed. Table 33.1 presents Kidney Injury score scale.

Conservative treatment is the choice for most of the patients. It has low rates of failure (1%), and it can save the kidneys and avoid iatrogenic lesions [2]. If intervention is indicated, nephrectomy, partial nephrectomy, renorrhaphy, urethral catheterization, and endovascular embolization are treatment options.

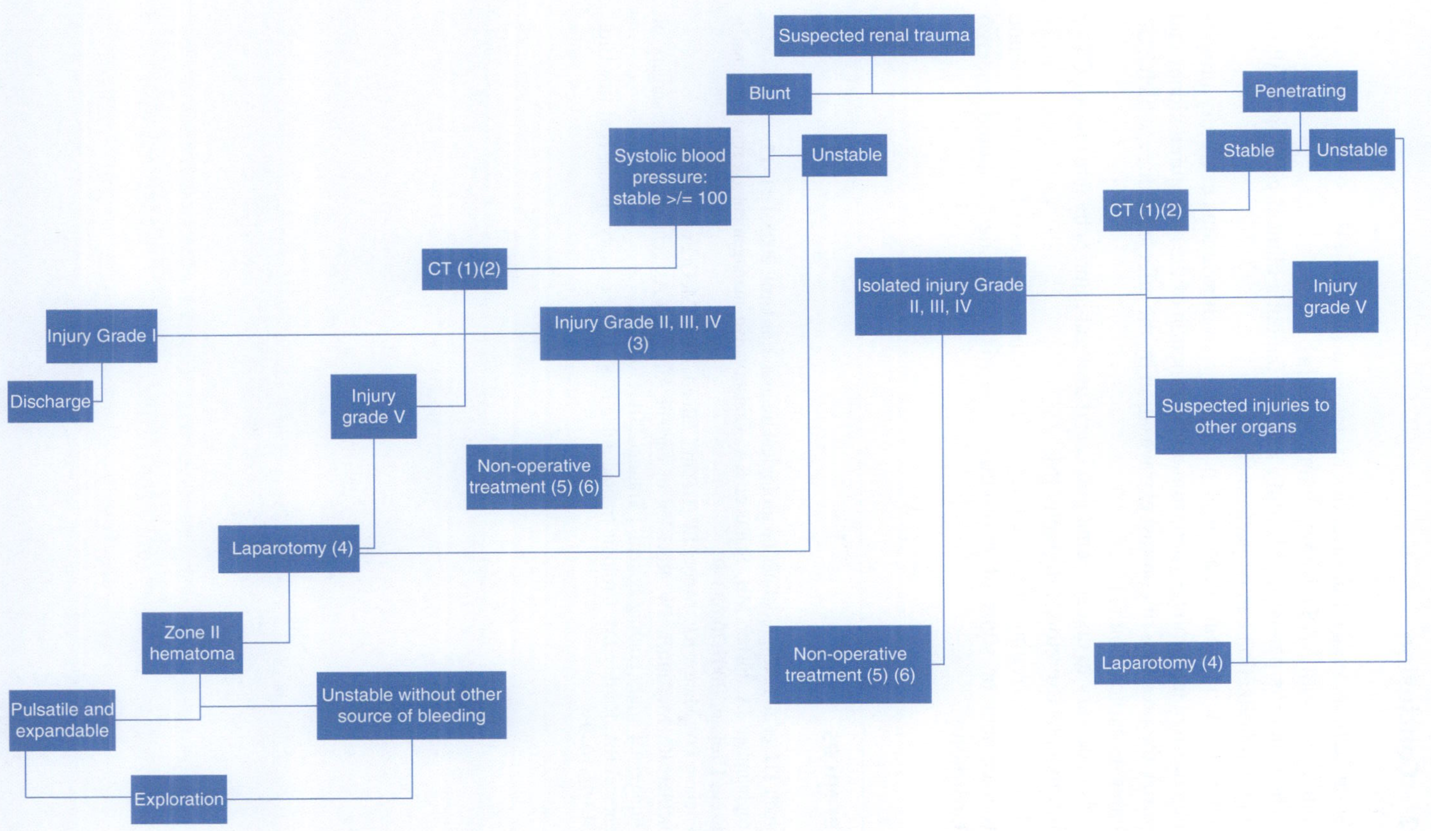

Suspected renal trauma
Blunt
Penetrating
Unstable
Stable
Unstable
Systolic blood pressure: stable >/= 100
CT (1)(2)
CT (1)(2)
Isolated injury Grade II, III, IV
Injury grade V
Injury Grade II, III, IV (3)
Injury Grade I
Discharge
Injury grade V
Suspected injuries to other organs
Non-operative treatment (5) (6)
Laparotomy (4)
Non-operative treatment (5) (6)
Laparotomy (4)
Zone II hematoma
Unstable without other source of bleeding
Pulsatile and expandable
Exploration

33.2 Conclusion

(1) Some authors suggest intravenous excretory urography [3].

(2) Table 33.1 with AAST Kidney Injury scale [4].

(3) When there is persisting bleeding and the patient's clinical conditions allow, angioembolization can be performed.

(4) There is the recommendation of performing an intravenous excretory urography during laparotomy to determinate the function of the noninjured kidney and verify the presence of contrast extravasation by the affected kidney, which indicates its exploration [1].

(5) It is necessary to discard renal pelvis and urethral injuries by late cuts of CT or intravenous excretory urography [5].

(6) If there is worsening of the hemodynamic status regardless of adequate volume replacement or signs of peritonitis or sepsis, the patients should undergo laparotomy.

References

1. Lynch TH, et al. EAU guidelines on urological trauma. Eur Urol. 2005;47:1–15.
2. Broghammer JA, Fisher MB, Santucci RA. Conservative management of renal trauma: a review. Urology. 2007;70:623–9.
3. Feliciano DV, Mattox KL, Moore EF. Trauma. 6th ed. EUA: McGraw Hill; 2008.
4. Buckley JC, McAninch JW. Revision of current American Association for the surgery of trauma renal injury grading system. J Trauma. 2011;70:35–7.
5. Santucci RA, Bartley JM. Urologic trauma guidelines: a 21st century update. Natl Rev Urol. 2010;7:510–9.

Urinary Tract Trauma

34

Eduardo Zanchet, Mateus Belotte,
Mariana F. Jucá Moscardi, Andrea Rachel Marcadis,
and Antonio Marttos

34.1 Introduction

The ureter is a thin and mobile structure which is protected in the retroperitoneum by the psoas muscle, spine, and pelvic bones [1]. Because of this relative protection, ureteral trauma corresponds to only 1% of all urinary trauma. The mechanism of ureteral trauma can be iatrogenic (75%), penetrating (18%), or blunt (7%), and is frequently associated with injuries to adjacent organs.

Only 43% of ureteral trauma cases present with hematuria, and therefore there are no pathognomonic signs of ureteral trauma. The diagnosis is usually performed by the visualization of contrast leakage into the retroperitoneum on helical computed tomography (CT) with late cuts. Excretory urography and retrograde pyelography are more precise exams, but they are not always able to be performed in patients with significant associated injuries. Often, the diagnosis is made by direct visualization during surgical exploration [2].

E. Zanchet · M. Belotte
Department of Surgery, Hospital do Trabalhador Trauma Center,
Federal University of Parana, Curitiba, Brazil

M. F. Jucá Moscardi (✉)
Telemedicine and Trauma Research, University of Miami, Ryder Trauma Center,
Miami, FL, USA

A. R. Marcadis
Department of Surgery, University of Miami, Miller School of Medicine, Jackson Memorial Hospital, Miami, FL, USA

A. Marttos
William Lehman Injury Research Center, Division of Trauma & Surgical Critical Care,
Dewitt Daughtry Department of Surgery, Leonard M. Miller School of Medicine Miami,
University of Miami, Miami, FL, USA

© Springer Nature Switzerland AG 2020
A. Nasr et al. (eds.), *The Trauma Golden Hour*,
https://doi.org/10.1007/978-3-030-26443-7_34

Table 34.1 AAST ureteral injuries scale

Grade	Type of injury	Description of injury
I	Hematoma	Contusion or hematoma without devascularization
II	Laceration	Transection <50%
III	Laceration	Transection ≥50%
IV	Laceration	Complete transection with <2 cm devascularization
V	Laceration	Avulsion with >2 cm of devascularization

Remarks: advance one grade for bilateral injuries up to grade III
Abbreviation: AAST: American Association for the Surgery of Trauma
Ref: [1]

Table 34.2 Treatment of ureteral injuries grade ≥ III

CT finding	Treatment
Superior third	Uretero-ureterostomy Transurethral ureterostomy Ureterocalicostomy
Middle third	Uretero-ureterostomy Transurethral ureterostomy Flap of Boari and ureteral reimplantation
Lower third	Flap of Boari and ureteral reimplantation Psychotic bladder or Blandy cystoplasty
Complete ureteral loss	Ileal interposition Autotransplant Both late

Abbreviation: *CT* computed tomography
Ref: [2]

The treatment of ureteral injuries is guided by the injury grade (Table 34.1) [1] and the site of the injury.

Grade I and II injuries can be treated by ureteral stent implantation or nephrostomy. Bigger lacerations can be treated as described in Table 34.2.

Surgical repair of ureteral injuries depends on some universally accepted principles: debridement of ureteral stumps, careful mobilization, use of absorbable sutures and ureteral stents, hermetic closure, as well as ureter isolation from associated injuries and retroperitoneum drainage [1].

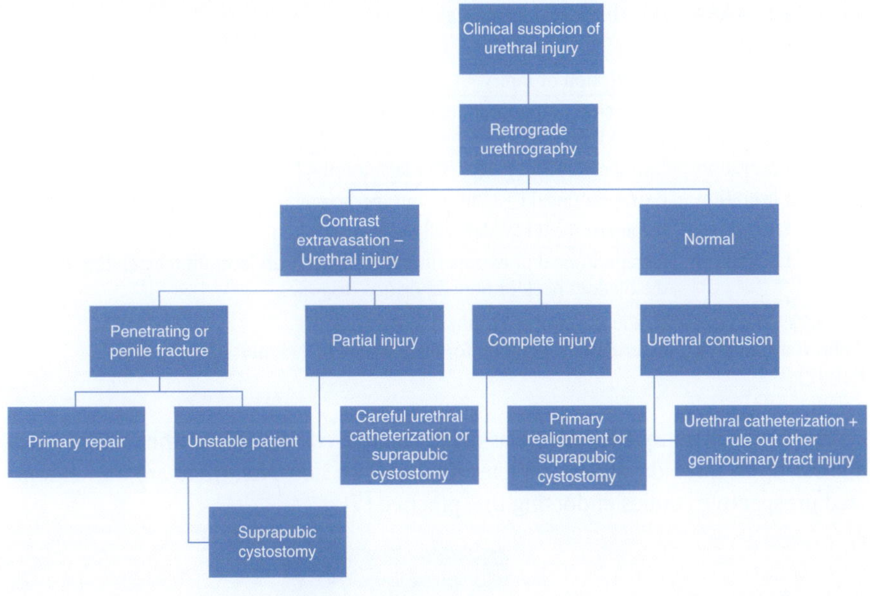

34.2 Bladder Trauma

Isolated blunt bladder trauma is rare, and normally it is associated with pelvic fractures. Blunt bladder injuries are usually extraperitoneal; however, intraperitoneal injuries can occur when there is blunt compression of the bladder dome when the bladder is full, causing a sudden increase of intravesicular pressure and consequent rupture [3]. Intraperitoneal bladder injury can also happen with penetrating trauma.

Hematuria (occurs in 95% of cases), abdominal pain, inability to urinate, gross scrotal or perineal hematoma, and abdominal distention are the most common signs and symptoms of bladder trauma. Diagnosis is generally made by retrograde cystography with 350 mL of contrast solution or by CT with the same amount of intravesical contrast [4]. Injuries are graded according to the scale described in Table 34.3 [2].

Extraperitoneal injuries are usually treated by closed-system urethral catheterization, with the catheter kept in place two weeks. Patients with penetrating injuries, intraperitoneal injuries, extraperitoneal injuries with intravesical bone spicules, rectal injuries, or those with open pelvic fractures require surgical exploration and correction [4].

Table 34.3 AAST urinary bladder injuries scale

Grade	Type of injury	Description of injury
I	Hematoma	Contusion, intramural hematoma
	Laceration	Partial thickness
II	Laceration	Extraperitoneal bladder wall laceration <2 cm
III	Laceration	Extraperitoneal ($\geq$2 cm) or intraperitoneal (<2 cm) bladder wall laceration
IV	Laceration	Intraperitoneal bladder wall laceration >2 cm.
V	Laceration	Intraperitoneal or extraperitoneal bladder wall laceration extending into the bladder neck or ureteral orifice (trigone)

Remarks: advance one grade for multiple injuries up to grade III
Abbreviation: AAST: American Association for the Surgery of Trauma
Ref: [2]

Prophylactic antibiotics have classically been used while the catheter is in place and for up to three days after catheter removal [4]; however, there are no randomized prospective studies endorsing this practice [7].

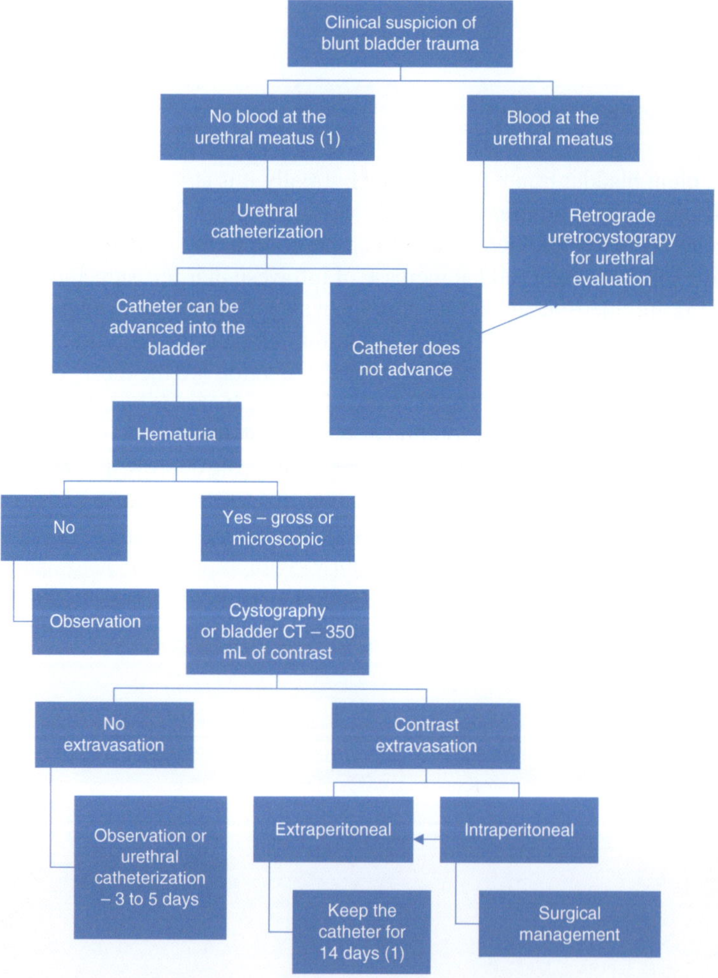

(1) Follow-up cystography: approximately 76–87% of the extraperitoneal injuries treated conservatively will heal in 10 days, and almost all will heal in 20 days. Therefore, a cystography is usually performed between the 10th and 14th day after injury. If there is no contrast extravasation, the urinary catheter is removed. If there is still extravasation, however, the catheter will be kept in place and a repeat cystography will be performed on day 21 [4].

34.3 Urethral Trauma

Urethral trauma is classified by the anatomical division of the anterior and posterior urethra. Posterior urethral injuries are usually associated with pelvic fractures, while anterior urethral injuries may be caused by direct trauma to the perineum, penetrating injuries, iatrogenic injuries, or sex-related injuries [6].

Understanding the clinical presentation is essential to the diagnosis of urethral injuries. The diagnosis should always be suspected in patients with pelvic fractures, perineal trauma, or penile trauma. The most common symptom is hematuria, and other common signs/symptoms are pain, penile hematoma, and difficulty urinating.

The diagnosis of urethral trauma is commonly made by retrograde urethrography, which can be performed using a 14- or 16-French Foley catheter with a 2-mL insufflated balloon at the navicular fossa [5]. It is possible to perform a careful urethral catheterization in a hemodynamically unstable patient; however, if this proves too difficult, the best option would be suprapubic cystostomy and posterior evaluation by uretrocistography [6].

The treatment of urethral injuries is based on the site and severity of the injury, which is defined by the AAST severity scale (Table 34.4). Conservative treatment with suprapubic cystotomy is generally the treatment of choice, as studies show that early manipulation of the urethra in urethral injuries may increase the incidence of erectile dysfunction and urinary incontinence [5].

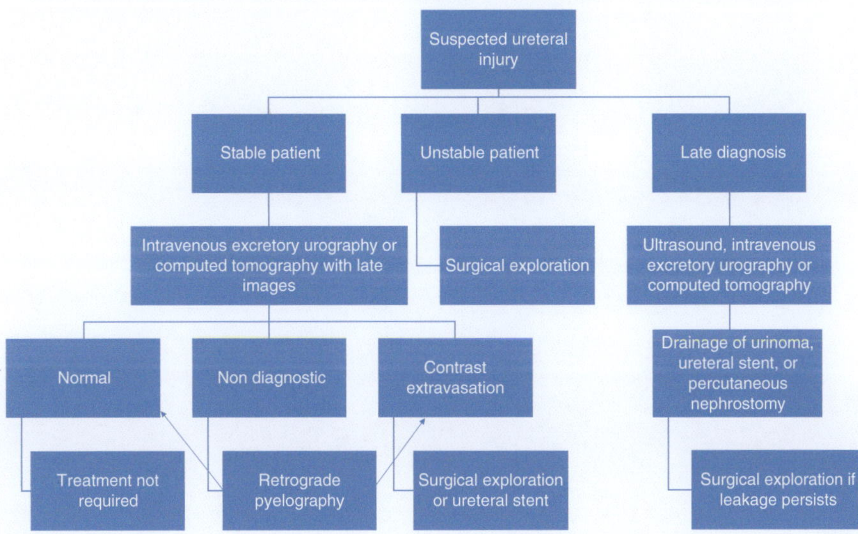

Table 34.4 AAST urethral injuries scale

Grade	Type of injury	Description of injury
I	Contusion	Blood at urethreal meatus; urethrography normal
II	Stretch injury	Elongation of urethra without extravasation on urethrography
III	Partial disruption	Extravasation of urethrography contract at injury site with visualization in the bladder
IV	Complete disruption	Extravasation of urethrography contrast at injury site without visualization in the bladder; <2 cm of uretheral separation
V	Complete disruption	Complete transection with ≥2 cm urethral separation, or extension into the prostate or vagina

Abbreviation: *AAST* American Association for the Surgery of Trauma

References

1. Pereira BMT, Ogilvie MP, Rodriguez JCG, Ryan ML, Peña D, Marttos AC, Pizano LR, McKenney MG. A review of ureteral injuries after external trauma. Scand J Trauma Resusc Emerg Med. 2010;18:6.
2. Lynch TH, Piñeiro LM, Plas E, Serafetinides E, Türkeri L, Santucci RA, Hohenfellner M. EAU guidelines on urological trauma. Eur Urol. 2005;47:1–15.
3. Shewakramani S, Reed KC. Genitourinary trauma. Emerg Med Clin N Am. 2011;29:501–18.
4. Santucci RA, Mcaninch JW. Bladder injuries: evaluation and management. Braz J Urol. 2000;26:408–14.
5. Rosenstein DI, Alsikafi NF. Diagnosis and classification of urethral injuries. Urol Clin N Am. 2006;33:73–85.
6. Piñeiro LM, Djakovic N, Plas E, Mor Y, Santucci RA, Serafetinidis E, Turkeri LN, .Hohenfellner M. EAU guidelines on urethral trauma, Eur Urol 57 (2010) 791–803
7. Tenke P, Kovacs B, Johansen TEB, Matsumoto T, Tambyahd PA, European NKG. Asian guidelines on management and prevention of catheter-associated urinary tract infections. Int J Antimicrob Agents. 2008;31S:S68–78.

Damage Control Surgery

35

Jéssica Romanelli Amorim de Souza, Phillipe Abreu,
Adonis Nasr, Flavio Saavedra Tomasich,
Antonio Marttos, and Iwan Collaço

35.1 Introduction

In the past few years, a lot has changed in the treatment of patients with life-threating conditions. The term "damage control surgery" was used for the first time by Rotondo in 1993. The author showed in his paper an improvement of 11–77% in mortality of patients with severe injuries submitted for the damage control surgery.

Damage control surgery (DCS) is an abbreviated laparotomy for patients who have life-threating bleeding, injuries, and septic sources. The procedure consists on hemorrhage control, by procedures like hemostasis, packing, clamping, and ligation; limits contamination by simple resections, primary suturation, closed absorbent systems, and external drainage; and leads to temporary abdominal closure as quickly as possible. The non-life-threatening injuries are delayed to a reoperation.

The main purpose of the damage control surgery is to prevent complications of the lethal triad: coagulopathy, acidosis, and hypothermia.

Damage control surgery was originally described by Rotondo as a three-phase technique but was then modified to a four-phase technique.

J. R. A. de Souza · P. Abreu (✉) · A. Nasr · F. Saavedra Tomasich
Iwan Collaço Trauma Research Group, Department of Surgery, Hospital do Trabalhador
Trauma Center, Federal University of Parana, Curitiba, Brazil

A. Marttos
William Lehman Injury Research Center, Division of Trauma & Surgical Critical Care,
Dewitt Daughtry Department of Surgery, Leonard M. Miller School of Medicine Miami,
University of Miami, Miami, FL, USA

I. Collaço
Department of Surgery, Hospital do Trabalhador Trauma Center, Federal University of
Parana, Curitiba, Brazil

© Springer Nature Switzerland AG 2020
A. Nasr et al. (eds.), *The Trauma Golden Hour*,
https://doi.org/10.1007/978-3-030-26443-7_35

- Stage 0: Recognition by the trauma team of the potential damage control beneficiaries. It is part of stage 0, the first step of resuscitation pre-hospitalar or initial evaluation stage. In this stage, rapid sequence of anesthesia and intubation is done, fluids given to restore normal vital parameters, with early warming and expedient transport to the operating room.
- Stage 1: Immediate exploratory laparotomy with quick control of hemorrhage, limit contamination and temporary abdominal closure.
- Stage 2: It is the resuscitation at intensive care unit (ICU) by physiological and biochemical stabilization. The main goal is to reverse the coagulopathy, acidosis, and hypothermia.
- Stage 3: Reoperation after the patient is stable and physiology has normalized. In the reoperation, the main goal is to repair all the injuries.

Main complications of damage control surgery are abdominal compartment syndrome, enterocutaneous fistulae and wound site problems, intraabdominal abscesses, multiple organs failure, and acute respiratory distress syndrome (Fig. 35.1).

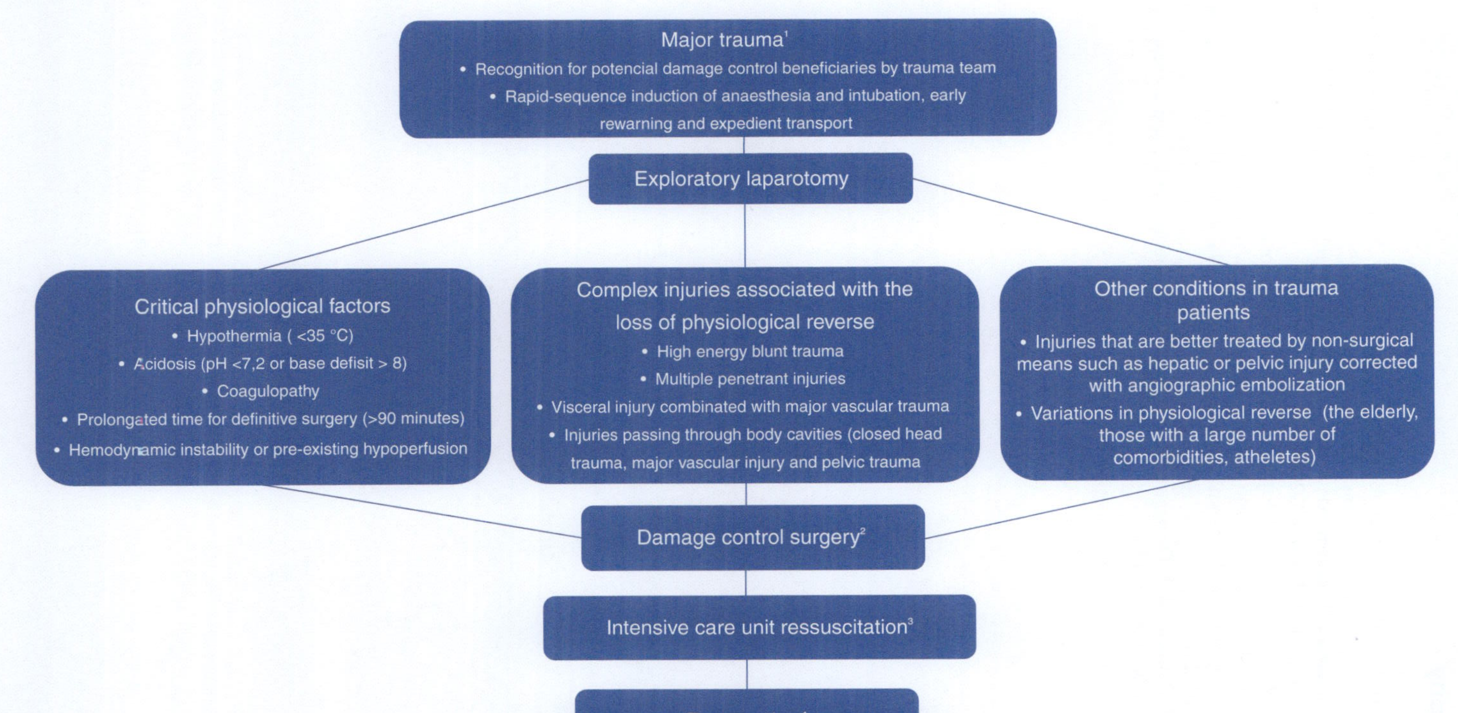

Fig. 35.1 Damage control surgery and its stages: (1) Stage 0; (2) Stage 1; (3) Stage 2; (4) Stage 3 [1–4]

Bibliography

1. Kanat BH, Bozan MB, Emir S et al. Damage control surgery. Actual problems of emergency abdominal surgery. 2016. DOI: https://doi.org/10.5772/64326.
2. Lamb CM, Macgoey P, Navarro AP, Brooks AJ. Damage control surgery in the era of damage control resuscitation. Br J Anaesth. 2014;113(2):242–9.
3. Mattox KL, Wall MJ, Jr, Tsai P. Chapter 24. Trauma Thoracotomy: Principles and Techniques. In: Mattox KL, Moore EE, Feliciano DV. eds. Trauma, 7e New York, NY: McGraw-Hill; 2013. http://accesssurgery.mhmedical.com/content.aspx?bookid=529§ionid=41077264. Accessed September 10, 2019.
4. Waibel BH, Rotondo MM. Damage control surgery: its evolution over the last 20 years. Rev Col Bras Cir. 2012;39(4):314–21.

Upper Extremity Trauma 36

José Marcos Lavrador Filho, Leonardo Dau,
Carlos Alberto Bidutte Cortez, Janaina de Oliveira Poy,
and Antonio Marttos

36.1 Introduction

Upper extremity traumas presented an exponential rise not only in quantity but also in complexity over the last years. Therefore, its initial approach when the patient arrives at the emergency room is very important to minimize posterior sequels of an unappropriated assessment.

Initial assessment (fast and objective) facilitates the treatment, improves the final outcome, decreases the sequels, and allows an early rehabilitation.

Most of the injuries occur at the same time (more than one associated injury). However, due to didactic purposes, we will divide the injuries into two groups. The first flowchart deals with soft tissue, nerve, and tendon injuries. The second and third flowcharts deal with several upper extremity fractures and dislocations.

J. M. L. Filho · L. Dau · C. A. B. Cortez
Department of Surgery, Hospital do Trabalhador Trauma Center, Federal University of Parana, Curitiba, Brazil

J. de Oliveira Poy
Faculdade de Ciências Médicas de Santos, Santos, São Paulo, Brazil

A. Marttos (✉)
William Lehman Injury Research Center, Division of Trauma & Surgical Critical Care, Dewitt Daughtry Department of Surgery, Leonard M. Miller School of Medicine Miami, University of Miami, Miami, FL, USA
e-mail: amarttos@med.miami.edu

© Springer Nature Switzerland AG 2020
A. Nasr et al. (eds.), *The Trauma Golden Hour*,
https://doi.org/10.1007/978-3-030-26443-7_36

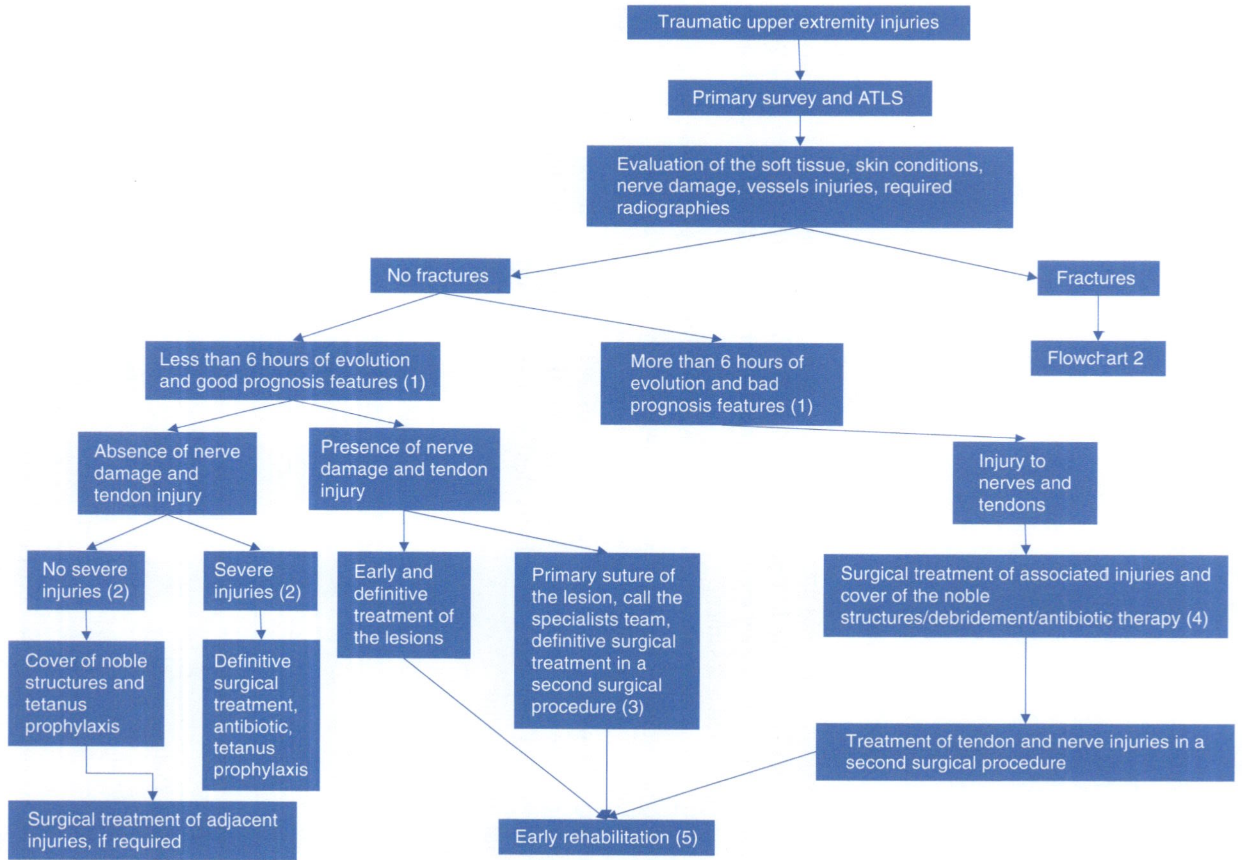

Traumatic upper extremity injuries
Primary survey and ATLS
Evaluation of the soft tissue, skin conditions, nerve damage, vessels injuries, required radiographies
No fractures
Fractures
Flowchart 2
Less than 6 hours of evolution and good prognosis features (1)
More than 6 hours of evolution and bad prognosis features (1)
Absence of nerve damage and tendon injury
Presence of nerve damage and tendon injury
Injury to nerves and tendons
No severe injuries (2)
Severe injuries (2)
Early and definitive treatment of the lesions
Primary suture of the lesion, call the specialists team, definitive surgical treatment in a second surgical procedure (3)
Surgical treatment of associated injuries and cover of the noble structures/debridement/antibiotic therapy (4)
Cover of noble structures and tetanus prophylaxis
Definitive surgical treatment, antibiotic, tetanus prophylaxis
Treatment of tendon and nerve injuries in a second surgical procedure
Surgical treatment of adjacent injuries, if required
Early rehabilitation (5)

(1) Good and bad prognosis: injuries with significant loss of skin cover, associated bone or vessel injuries, more than 6 hours of evolution, and loss of segments (nerves and tendons).
(2) Severe injuries: soft tissue conditions, bone exposure, and deformities or injuries that could compromise the limb viability.
(3) Second intervention for definitive care: can be performed until 14 days after the injury, preferably a termino-terminal nonabsorbable suture or using graft/transference when there is no possibility of direct reconstruction.
(4) Noble structures: bones, tendons, nerves.
(5) Rehabilitation: physiotherapy/occupational therapy.

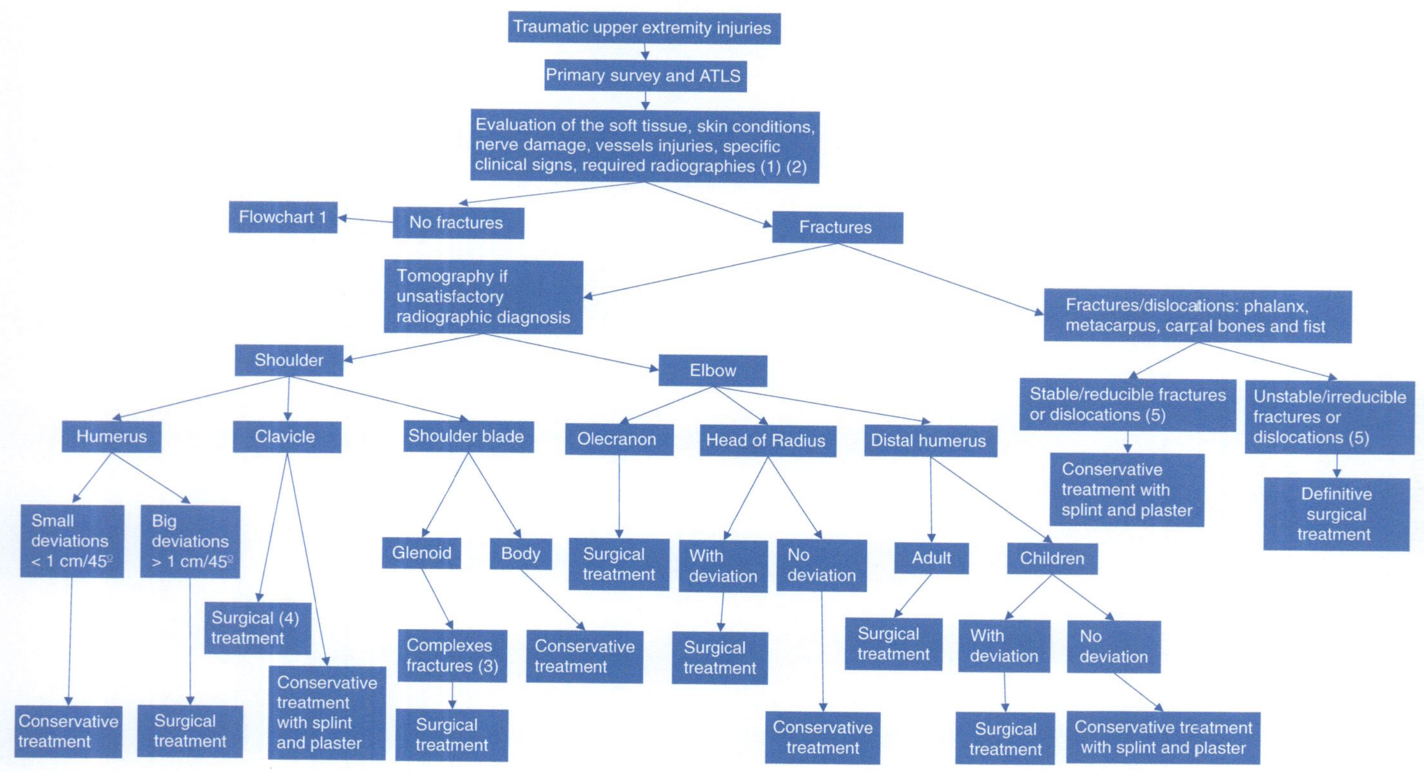

Traumatic upper extremity injuries
Primary survey and ATLS
Evaluation of the soft tissue, skin conditions, nerve damage, vessels injuries, specific clinical signs, required radiographies (1) (2)
Flowchart 1
No fractures
Fractures
Tomography if unsatisfactory radiographic diagnosis
Fractures/dislocations: phalanx, metacarpus, carpal bones and fist
Stable/reducible fractures or dislocations (5)
Unstable/irreducible fractures or dislocations (5)
Conservative treatment with splint and plaster
Definitive surgical treatment
Shoulder
Elbow
Humerus
Clavicle
Shoulder blade
Olecranon
Head of Radius
Distal humerus
Small deviations < 1 cm/45°
Big deviations > 1 cm/45°
Surgical (4) treatment
Glenoid
Body
Surgical treatment
With deviation
No deviation
Adult
Children
Conservative treatment
Surgical treatment
Conservative treatment with splint and plaster
Complexes fractures (3)
Conservative treatment
Surgical treatment
Surgical treatment
Surgical treatment
With deviation
No deviation
Conservative treatment
Surgical treatment
Conservative treatment with splint and plaster

(1) Specific clinical signs: local hematomas, signs of shoulder dislocation, signs of shoulder instability.
(2) Radiographic incidences: true anterior-posterior, Neer profile, and axillary. Bilateral Zanca, Stryker incidence.
(3) Surgical treatment indications in glenoid fracture: neck fractures with shortening bigger than 1 cm or varus deviation bigger than 40°, cavitation fractures if deviation is bigger than 5 mm or fractures of the edge causing instability.
(4) Surgical treatment indications in clavicle fracture: shortening bigger than 2 cm and diastasis bigger than 1 cm.
(5) Fractures instability criteria [1]:
    (a) Metaphyseal comminution (multifragmented fractures).
    (b) Joint fractures.
    (c) Dorsal or volar deviations > 20°.
    (d) Bone shortening > 5 mm.
    (e) Associated ulna fracture.
    (f) Osteoporosis (or age > 60 years).
(6) Position intrinsic-plus: functional position of the fist/hand, where the fist has a dorsal deviation of 30°, the metacarpal phalanges with flexion of 70–90°, and the interphalangeal in complete extension of 0° [2–8].

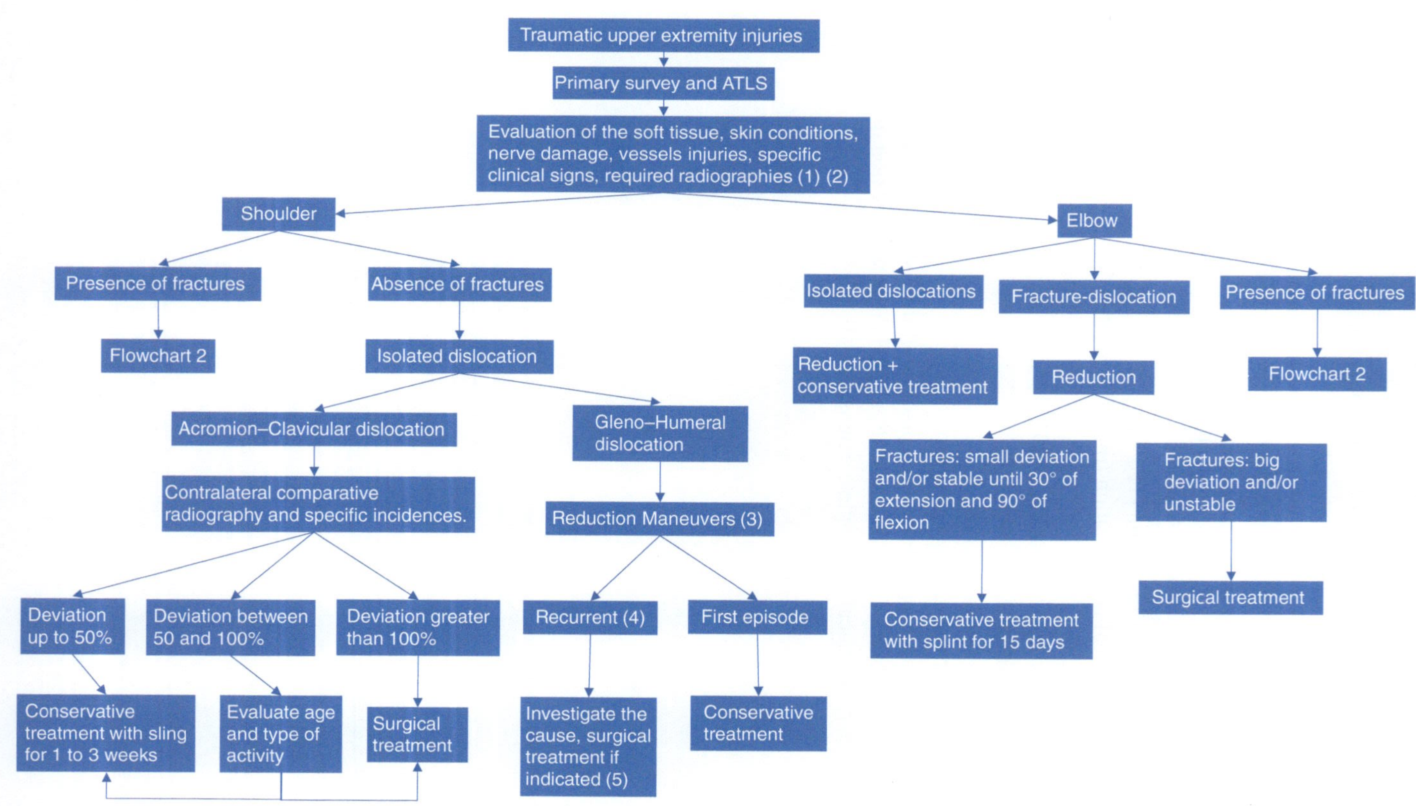

Traumatic upper extremity injuries
Primary survey and ATLS
Evaluation of the soft tissue, skin conditions, nerve damage, vessels injuries, specific clinical signs, required radiographies (1) (2)
Shoulder
Elbow
Presence of fractures
Absence of fractures
Isolated dislocations
Fracture-dislocation
Presence of fractures
Flowchart 2
Isolated dislocation
Reduction + conservative treatment
Reduction
Flowchart 2
Acromion–Clavicular dislocation
Gleno–Humeral dislocation
Fractures: small deviation and/or stable until 30° of extension and 90° of flexion
Fractures: big deviation and/or unstable
Contralateral comparative radiography and specific incidences.
Reduction Maneuvers (3)
Conservative treatment with splint for 15 days
Surgical treatment
Deviation up to 50%
Deviation between 50 and 100%
Deviation greater than 100%
Recurrent (4)
First episode
Conservative treatment with sling for 1 to 3 weeks
Evaluate age and type of activity
Surgical treatment
Investigate the cause, surgical treatment if indicated (5)
Conservative treatment

(1) Specific clinical signs: local hematomas, signs of dislocation, signs of instability.
(2) Radiographic incidences: true anterior-posterior, Neer profile, and axillary. Bilateral Zanca, Stryker incidence.
(3) Reduction maneuvers, traction/counter traction maneuvers, lateral traction/counter traction, Stimson method, Much method, Hippocrates method, Kocher method.
(4) Surgical indication: irreducibility, young patients, recurrent dislocation, interposition of soft tissues making it irreducible, rotator cuff lesions, and glenoid edge fractures.

Bibliography

1. Lafontaine M, Hardy D, Delince P. Stability assessment of distal radius fractures. Injury. 1989;20(4):208–10.
2. Wolfe SW, Hotchkiss RN, Pederson WC, Kozin SH. Green's operative hand surgery. 6ª ed. Philadelphia: Elsevier; 2011.
3. Pardini A, Freitas A. Traumatismos da mão, 4ª ed. Rio de Janeiro, RJ: Medbook; 2008.
4. Trumble TE, Budoff JE, Cornwall R. Hand, elbow & shoulder, core knowledge in orthopaedics. Philadelphia: Mosby Elsevier; 2006.
5. Reis FB. Fraturas, 2ª ed. Sao Paulo, SP: Atheneu; 2007.
6. Herbert S, Xavier R. Princípios em ortopedia, 4ª ed. Porto Alegre, RS: Artmed; 2009.
7. Rockwood CA Jr, Matsen FA III, Wirth MA, Lippitt SB. The shoulder. 4ª ed. Philadelphia: Saunders; 2009.
8. Morrey BF, Sanches-Sotelo J. The elbow and its disorders. 4ª ed. Philadelphia: Saunders; 2009.

Lower Extremity Injuries

37

Haiana Lopes Cavalheiro, Christiano Saliba Uliana,
Marcello Zaia Oliveira, Mariana F. Jucá Moscardi,
and Antonio Marttos

37.1 Introduction

In this chapter, we describe the conduct on the main injuries of the lower limb. Remember that the conducts mentioned here can be individualized according to the bone quality, type of fracture, chronological and biological age, and trauma energy.

Every patient victim of a lower extremity trauma should undergo a careful evaluation of the extremities. This evaluation includes palpation of the femoral, popliteal, pedal, and posterior tibial pulses. And also the evaluation of the sensibility of each dermatome and motility of each nerve root. This evaluation should be made after the end of the primary survey (ABCDE) and if the patient shows tendency to normalize his/her vital functions. The extremities evaluation should be repeated in a short time period, especially if the patient is already hemodynamically stable.

H. L. Cavalheiro
Iwan Collaço Trauma Research Group, Department of Surgery, Hospital do Trabalhador Trauma Center, Federal University of Parana, Curitiba, Brazil

C. S. Uliana · M. Z. Oliveira
Department of Surgery, Hospital do Trabalhador Trauma Center, Federal University of Parana, Curitiba, Brazil

M. F. Jucá Moscardi (✉)
Telemedicine and Trauma Research, University of Miami, Ryder Trauma Center, Miami, FL, USA

A. Marttos
William Lehman Injury Research Center, Division of Trauma & Surgical Critical Care, Dewitt Daughtry Department of Surgery, Leonard M. Miller School of Medicine Miami, University of Miami, Miami, FL, USA

© Springer Nature Switzerland AG 2020
A. Nasr et al. (eds.), *The Trauma Golden Hour*,
https://doi.org/10.1007/978-3-030-26443-7_37

Flowchart 1

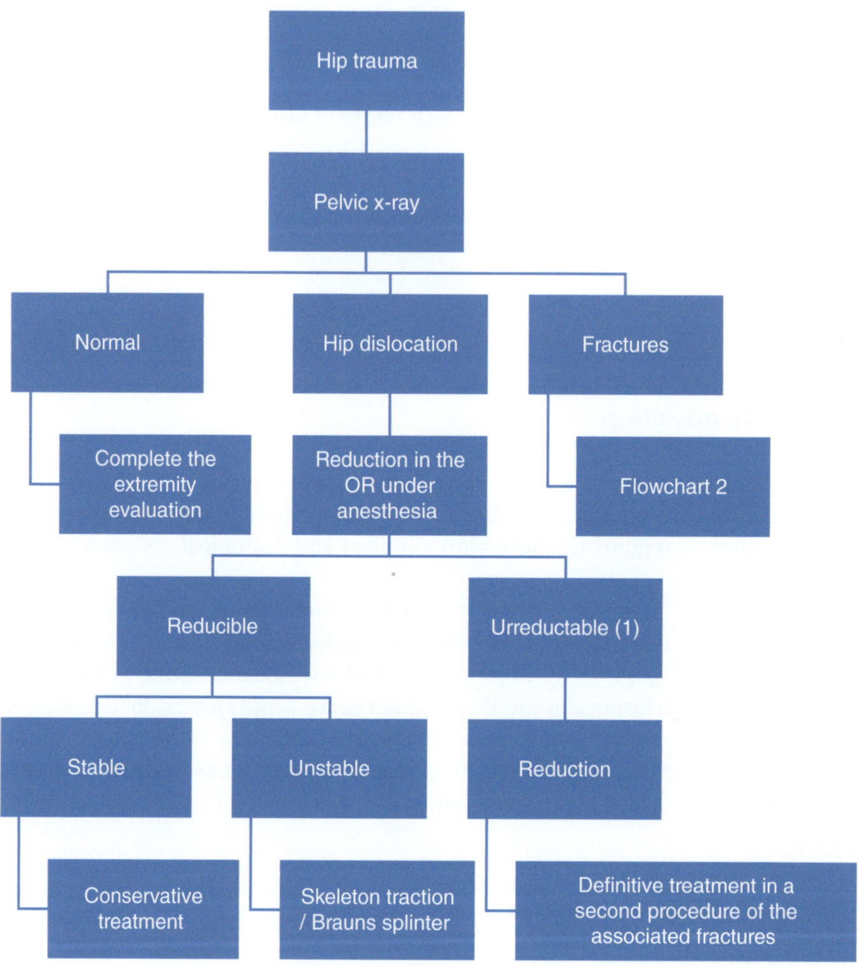

(1) Frequently associated with fracture of the femoral head and the acetabulum.

Flowchart 2

Pelvic trauma
Subtrochanteric
Transtrochanteric
Neck
Acetabulum
Polytrauma
Isolated trauma
External fixation
Definitive treatment in a second surgery
Analgesia
Fixation with internal synthesis (< 48 hours)
1.3.1. Early surgical treatment (< 48 hours) (1)
Patient > 75 years
Patient < 65 years
Deviation
No deviation
Arthroplasty
Anatomical reduction and surgical fixation
Anatomical reduction and surgical fixation
No dislocation
Hip dislocation
Analgesia
Flowchart 1 box 2.2
Latte Surgical treatment
Conservative treatment

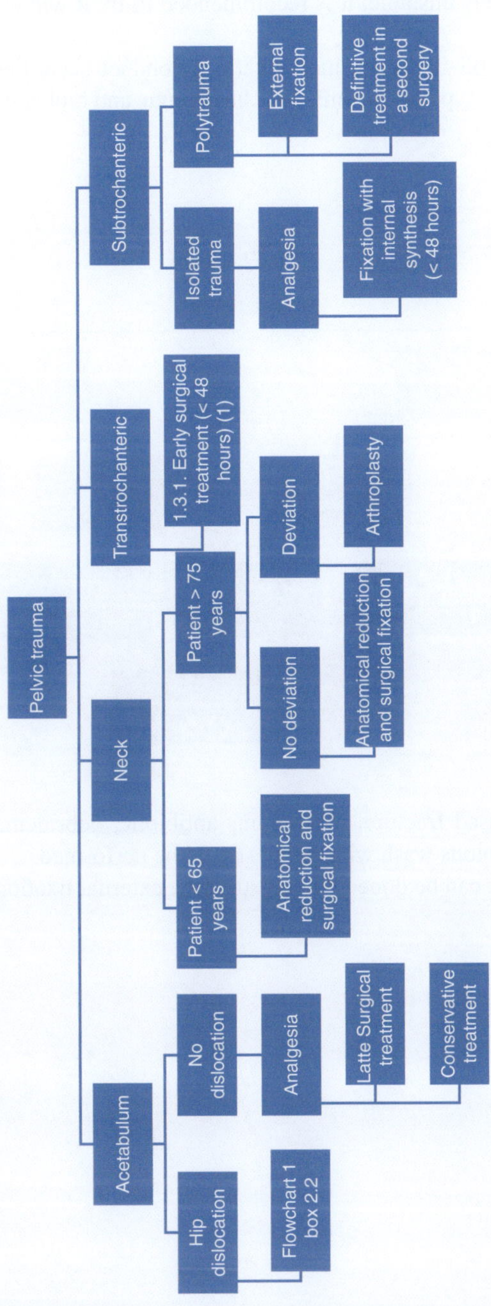

(1) If the fracture is stable, it is recommended to fix it with sliding plate and screw. If the fracture is unstable, it is recommended to fix it with a cephalo-medullar stem.
(2) Patients with 65–75 years: individualized conduct according to bone quality, trauma energy, type of fracture, and chronologic and biologic age of the patient.

Flowchart 3

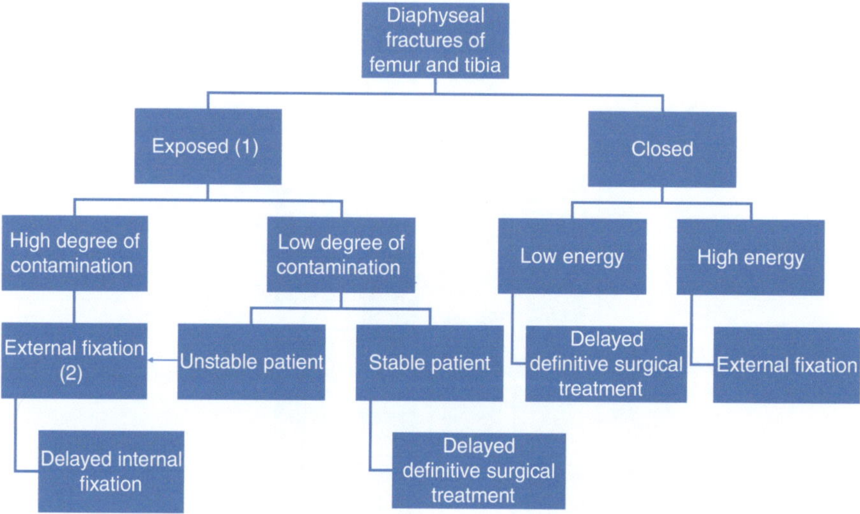

(1) In every exposed fracture, intravenous antibiotic, debridement of devitalized tissue, and copious wash with saline should be performed.
(2) A second look can be done 48 hours after the external fixation for cleaning and debridement

Flowchart 4

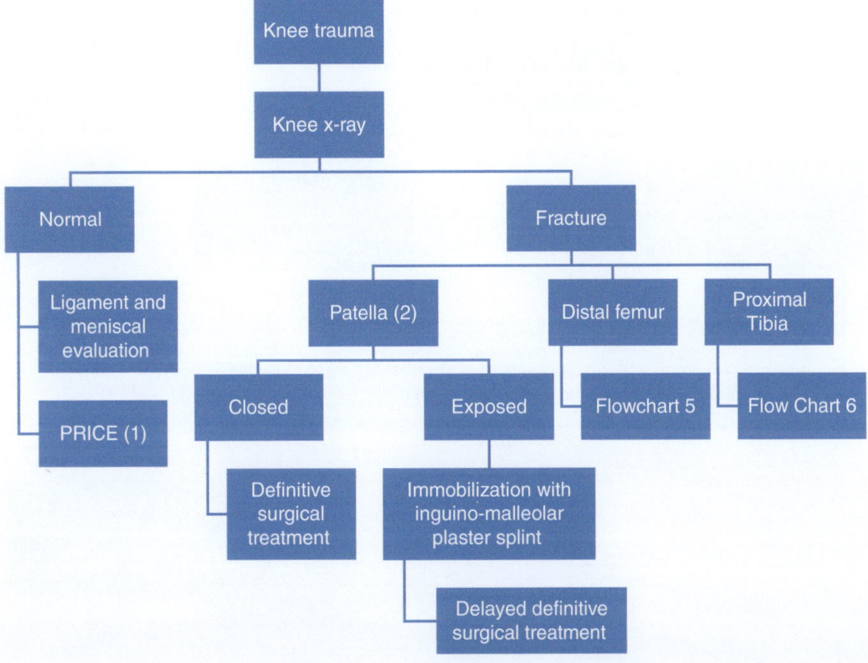

(1) Protection, resting, limb elevation, cold compress, and immobilization.
(2) Perform an axial X-ray of the patella.

Flowchart 5

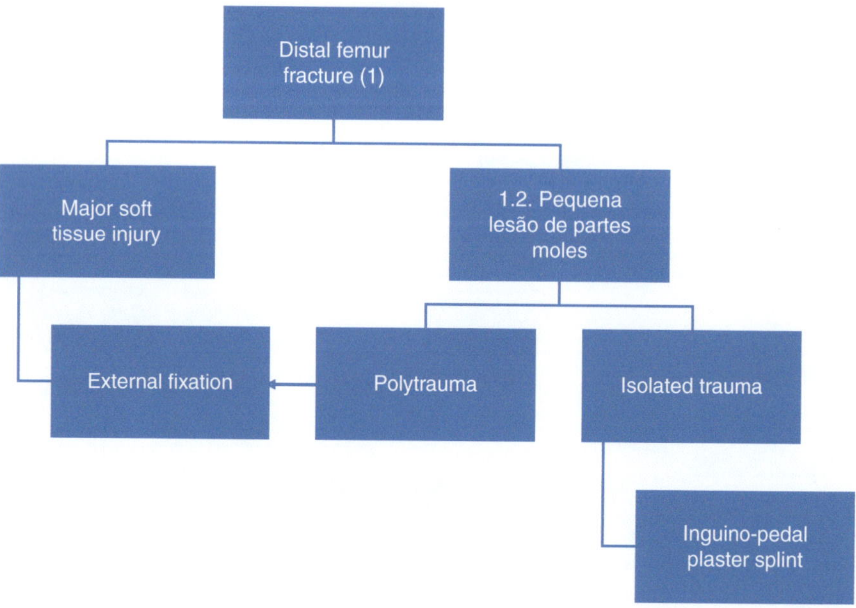

(1) Distal femur fractures can be articular or extra-articular. This differentiation is important in articular fractures, and an evaluation by computed tomography is recommended.

Flowchart 6

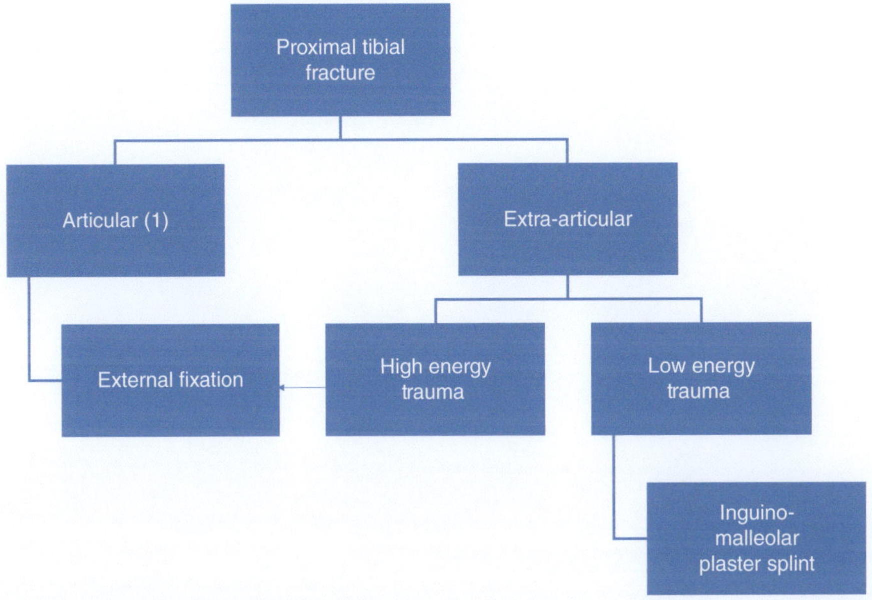

(1) In articular fractures, an evaluation by computed tomography should be done.

Bibliography

1. Chapter 45 – Lesões dos joelhos. Fraturas em adultos, Rockwood e Green, 5th ed., p. 1843
2. Canale ST ed., Chapter 43 – Lesões do Joelho, 10th ed., Cirurgia ortopédica de Campbell, p. 2165
3. Ruedi TP, Buckley RE, Moran CG. Princípios do tratamento de fraturas. 2nd ed., 1st vol – Princípios, 2nd vol – Fraturas Específicas

Burn Care

38

Bruna Arcoverde Abbott, Maykon Martins de Souza,
Renato da Silva Freitas, Ana Luisa Bettega,
and Carl Ivan Schulman

38.1 Introduction

Burn injury is a serious health problem that can affect any social group and age range, producing countless victims worldwide. In Brazil, burn is the second largest cause of death in children, and is most prevalent at the extremes of age. The major causes of severe burn injury in younger patients are liquid scalds. Flame burns are more common in adult patients and also responsible for most deaths.

In the last decades, there was a dramatic improvement in mortality after massive burns, which is associated with better resuscitation, improvements in wound coverage by early excision and grafting, better support of the hypermetabolic response, early nutritional support, more appropriate control of infection, and improved treatment of inhalation injuries.

There are six causal categories of burns: fire, scald, contact, chemical, electrical, and radiation. Flame, scald, and contact burns cause cellular damage by the transfer of energy that induces coagulative necrosis, while chemical and electrical burns cause direct damage to cellular membranes. The skin acts like a barrier, but after the source of burn is removed, the response of local tissues can lead to further injury. The necrotic area of the burn is termed the "zone of coagulation," and the surrounding area (that has a moderate degree of injury that initially causes a decrease in

B. A. Abbott · M. M. de Souza · A. L. Bettega (✉)
Iwan Collaço Trauma Research Group, Department of Surgery, Hospital do Trabalhador
Trauma Center, Federal University of Parana, Curitiba, Brazil

R. da Silva Freitas
Division of Plastic Surgery, Department of Surgery, Hospital do Trabalhador Trauma Center,
Federal University of Parana, Curitiba, Brazil

C. I. Schulman
Division of Trauma Surgery & Critical Care, DeWitt Daughtry Family Department of
Surgery, Miller School of Medicine, University of Miami, Miami, FL, USA

© Springer Nature Switzerland AG 2020
A. Nasr et al. (eds.), *The Trauma Golden Hour*,
https://doi.org/10.1007/978-3-030-26443-7_38

tissue perfusion) is the "zone of stasis." The "zone of hyperemia" is formed as a result of vasodilation from inflammation surrounding the burn wound and contains viable tissue.

38.2 Inflammatory Response

Significant burn can lead to hypermetabolic response and massive release of inflammatory mediators in the wound. The hypermetabolism is mediated by increases in circulation levels of catabolic hormones (catecholamines, cortisol, and glucagon) and is associated with alterations in blood serum glucose, hyperdynamic cardiovascular response, increased energy expenditure, loss of lean body mass and body weight, accelerated breakdown of glycogen and protein, lipolysis, and immune depression. Many mediators have been proposed to explain the changes in vascular permeability such as catecholamines, histamine, bradykinin, vasoactive amines, leukotrienes, and activated complement. Also, aggregated platelets release serotonin that improves the formation of edema. Another important mediator is thromboxane A2, which is a potent vasoconstrictor leading to platelet aggregation and contributing to expansion of the zone of stasis.

Major burn injury results in multiple organ dysfunction, including cardiac and pulmonary effects, decrease in renal blood flow and fall in glomerular filtration rate, hepatic steatosis due to increased peripheral lipolysis, and generalized impairment in host defenses that leads to increased susceptibility to infections. All burn-related metabolic responses last more than 2 years post-burn.

38.3 Initial Care

Since every burn victim should be considered as a trauma victim, the initial assessment should be fast and objective following clear rules observing basically the following parameters: age of the patient, affected site of the body, burn body surface area and identifying the causative agent of the lesion, other associated traumas, comorbidities, social conditions, and depth of burns.

The patient should be removed from the source of the burn to stop burning process, and clothing and jewelry should be immediately removed. Then, the patient should be placed on sterile or clean sheets; cold water and ice are not recommended since they can harm by inducing hypothermia.

Regarding the depth of the lesion, they can be classified as follows: first degree which comprises only the epidermis, second degree reaching also partially the dermis, and third degree in which injuries have spread to the entire thickness of the dermis. To calculate the burn surface area, the patient's own hand rule, which represents approximately 1% of the body area, or the "rule of nines," can be used.

After the classification of the patient through the parameters described above, a coordinated order of steps is required to perform a correct risk stratification which will allow evaluating if hospitalization or outpatient treatment is needed or if the patient needs to be transferred to a specialized burn care center. For that, we elaborate the following practical and objective algorithm:

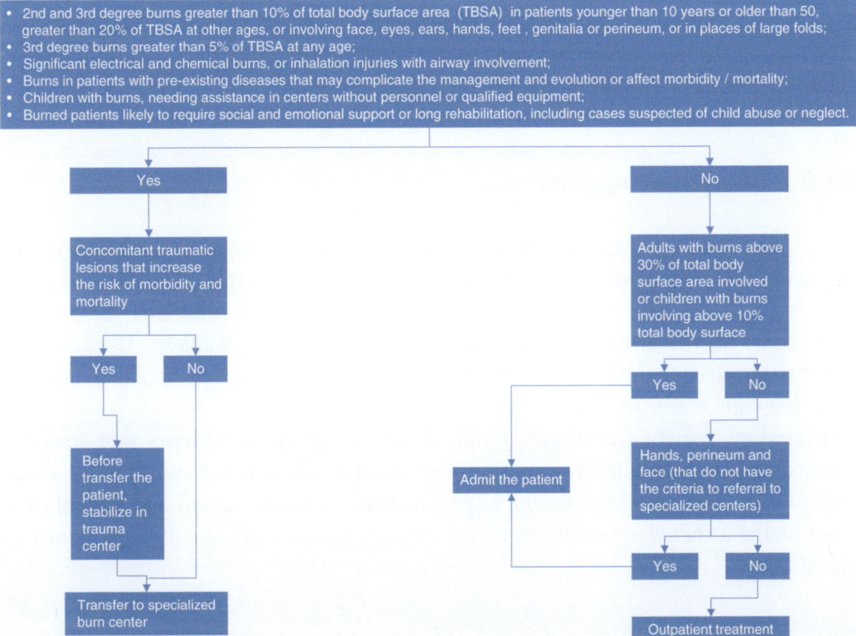

It is important to evaluate the airway once airway obstruction due to inhalation injury or edema can be present and indicate immediate treatment with intubation. Arterial blood gas and carboxyhemoglobin levels should be obtained when inhalation injury is suspected. Noninvasive measurement of blood pressure may be difficult in patients with burned extremities, so an arterial line may be necessary to monitor the blood pressure during transfer or resuscitation. The insertion of a femoral arterial line may be more appropriate.

The best intravenous access can be obtained with short large-bore peripheral catheters through unburned skin. Other options are central venous lines or intraosseous access. Lactated Ringer's solution without dextrose is the fluid of choice except in children less than 2 years of age. Infants should receive some 5% dextrose in intravenous solutions to prevent hypoglycemia because they have limited glycogen stores. The initial rate can be rapidly estimated by multiplying the estimated total body surface area (TBSA) burned by the weight in kilograms, which is divided by 4 to get an hourly rate for the first 8 hours (Parkland formula). Children have a larger body surface area relative to their weight compared to adults and generally have grater fluid needs during resuscitation. The Galveston formula for children based on body surface area uses 5000 ml/m^2 TBSA burned for resuscitation + 1500 ml/m^2 TBSA for maintenance in the first 24 hours. Over-resuscitation can be prevented by monitoring urine output, which should be maintained at 0.5 ml/kg/h in adults and 1.0 ml/kg/h in children.

38.4 Chemical Burns

In chemical burns, it is necessary to prompt treatment to minimize tissue damage and the area should be copiously irrigated with water. Attempts at neutralization of either acidic or basic solutions can result in heat production and extend the injury. Chemical burns are typically deeper than that appears.

38.5 Electrical Injuries

They may be mostly internal, affecting nerves, blood vessels, and muscle, and sparing skin, except at the contact point of the electrical current. Electrical injuries require vigorous intravenous resuscitation (urine output maintained at greater than 1 ml/kg/h) and attention to myoglobinuria from muscle damage. If necessary, administration of mannitol to increase renal tubular flow and bicarbonate to alkalize the urine can be considered.

Important burns in extremities may lead to generalized edema that impedes venous outflow and will have a tourniquet effect on the arterial inflow to the distal beds. The release of a burn eschar is performed by making lateral and medial incisions on the affected extremity using the electrocautery to release the obstruction to blood flow.

38.6 Wound Care

Once the extent and depth of the wounds have been assessed and the wounds have been thoroughly cleaned and debrided, the management phase begins. The choice of dressing should be individualized. First-degree burns require no dressing and can be treated with lotion to keep the skin moist. Second-degree burns can be treated with an antibiotic ointment and covered with gauze under elastic wraps. Alternatively, the wounds can be covered with a temporary biologic or synthetic covering to close the wound, including biological materials such as allograft skin, porcine xenograft skin, human amniotic membranes, and synthetic materials and silver-impregnated dressings.

38.7 Surgical Treatment

Most surgeons practice early excision and skin graft due to benefit over serial debridements in terms of survival, blood loss, and length of hospitalization. After the excision, the wound must be covered with autograft skin or another covering. The recommendation is to perform the excision immediately after stabilization of the patient, and once blood loss diminishes, the operation can be performed the first day after injury.

Skin graft loss after an operation is typically due to the presence of infection, fluid collection under the graft, shearing forces that disrupt the adhered graft, or an inadequate excision of the wound bed.

38.8 Control of Infection

The topical antibiotics can be salves or soaks. Salves are generally applied once or twice a day directly to the wound with dressings placed over them, and include 8.5% mafenide acetate, 1% silver sulfadiazine, polymyxin B, neomycin, bacitracin, and mupirocin. Soaks with antimicrobial solutions are generally poured into dressings on the wound, and include 0.5% silver nitrate solution, 0.025% sodium hypochlorite, 5% acetic acid, and 5% mafenide acetate solution.

Besides, perioperative systemic antimicrobials are useful in decreasing sepsis in the burn wound. Choosing the antimicrobial is important to cover *S. aureus* and *Pseudomonas* sp. that are prevalent in wounds.

Bibliography

1. Moore E, Feliciano D, Mattox K. Trauma. 8th ed. New York: McGraw-Hill Education; 2017. p. 945–55.
2. Warden GD, et al. Fluid resuscitation and early management. In: Herndon DN, editor. Total burn care. 4th ed. London: Saunders; 2012. p. 115–25.
3. Williams FN, Jeschke MG, Chinkes DL, Suman OF, Branski LK, Herndon DN. Modulation of the post-burn hypermetabolic response to trauma: temperature, nutrition, and drugs. J Am Coll Surg. 2009;208:489–502.
4. Townsend C, Beauchamp D. Sabiston. Tratado de cirurgia, vol. 1. 19a ed: Elsevier; 2014. p. 521–46.
5. Gomes D, Serra M, Pellon M. Queimaduras. Editora Revinter Ltda, 1995.

Trauma in Pregnancy

Denise Magalhães Machado, Seung Hoon Shin,
Marcos Takimura, Acácia Maria Fávaro Nasr,
Ana Luisa Bettega, and Edward B. Lineen

39.1 Introduction

Trauma is the main cause of nonobstetric death in pregnancy with an overall prevalence of 6–7%. It is said that fetal mortality in a severe trauma reaches up to 61%, and if there is maternal shock, to 80% [1]. The most common cause is car accident with 55%, and it is also the main cause of traumatic fetal death (82%) [2].

Although the initial assessment and management priorities for resuscitation of injured pregnant patients are the same as that for nonpregnant patients, the specific anatomic and physiologic changes during the pregnancy may alter the response to injury, so a modified approach is needed. And the main principle guiding therapy must be that resuscitating the mother will resuscitate the fetus. Multidisciplinary team approach including an obstetrician is essential.

In the trauma resuscitation bay, patients ≥20 weeks of gestational age (GA) should be in left lateral position (right side up) to avoid IVC compression [3]. The pregnant patients have a greater risk for airway management and difficult intubation than nonpregnant patients. Early intubation [3] with a smaller size of

D. M. Machado · A. L. Bettega (✉)
Iwan Collaço Trauma Research Group, Department of Surgery, Hospital do Trabalhador
Trauma Center, Federal University of Parana, Curitiba, Brazil

S. H. Shin
Ryder Trauma Center – Jackson Health System, Miami, FL, USA

Miller School of Medicine, University of Miami, Miami, FL, USA

M. Takimura · A. M. F. Nasr
Department of Obstetrics and Gynecology, Hospital do Trabalhador Trauma Center,
Federal University of Parana, Curitiba, Brazil

E. B. Lineen
Division of Trauma Surgery & Critical Care, DeWitt Daughtry Family Department of
Surgery, Miller School of Medicine, University of Miami, Miami, FL, USA

© Springer Nature Switzerland AG 2020
A. Nasr et al. (eds.), *The Trauma Golden Hour*,
https://doi.org/10.1007/978-3-030-26443-7_39

endotracheal tubes [4] are recommended. NG tubes should be considered in patients with altered mental status due to the risk of aspiration [5].

Routine supplemental oxygen is mandated to keep maternal oxygen saturation >95% [3] because of decreased functional residual capacity from maternal anatomical change and marked increases in oxygen consumption. Insertion of the thoracostomy tube should be one or two intercostal spaces higher than usual [3, 5].

Aggressive volume resuscitation is encouraged even for normotensive patients because pregnant patients' physiologic changes may mask signs of hypovolemia. When the signs of shock appear, fetal mortality rate increases to 85%. The uteroplacental flow insufficiency could happen before the signs of maternal shock. Also, the uteroplacental vasculature is highly responsive to vasopressors. In case of maternal hypotension, vasopressors should be avoided unless the patient is unresponsive to volume replacement [3].

Regarding the secondary survey, in addition to the routine ATLS assessment, obstetrical aspects need to be assessed, which are obstetric history, vaginal and rectal exam, estimation of GA, fetal heart monitoring, and so on. Abdominal examination of pregnant patients is less informative in ruling out major organ injury and further investigation should be conducted [6]. FAST and DPL are useful tools to evaluate intraperitoneal injury and their sensitivities are similar to one of nonpregnant patients.

Diagnostic studies should not be withheld out of concern for fetal radiation exposure. Exposure of the fetus <5–10 rad causes no significant increase in the risk of congenital malformation, intrauterine growth retardation, or miscarriage [1]. It is preferable to perform a single CT scan with iodinated contrast rather than perform multiple suboptimal studies without contrast [7].

All pregnant trauma patients of >20 weeks of GA require cardiotocographic (CTG) monitoring for minimum 6 hours [1]. Traumatic placental injury can result in feto-maternal hemorrhage (FMH) in about 10–30% of pregnant trauma patients [5]. It could happen after 12 weeks of GA. One dose of anti-D IgG should be given to all Rh-negative pregnant trauma patients within 72 hours to prevent maternal sensitization [8]. One dose (300 mcg) covers 30 ml of fetal blood in maternal circulation. The Kleihauer–Betke test can be useful to determine whether the additional dose anti-D IgG is needed [8].

Placental abruption is the leading cause of fetal death following trauma accounting for 50–70% of all trauma-related fetal loses [7]. Vaginal bleeding showed 80% of cases. Ultrasound (US) may detect abruption, but it has high false-negative rate (50–80%) [9]. Abruption may follow even minor trauma and requires high index of suspicion to detect. CTG is the most useful method to detect clinically silent cases. Occult or concealed abruption may lead to major maternal bleeding and consumption coagulopathy. Significant abruption requires urgent delivery by cesarean section (c-section).

In the case of maternal cardiac arrest, follow ATLS guidelines and defibrillate and/or use ACLS drugs as indicated. Consider perimortem c-section in ED if ≥20 weeks of GA and no response to effective CPR after 4 minutes [10].

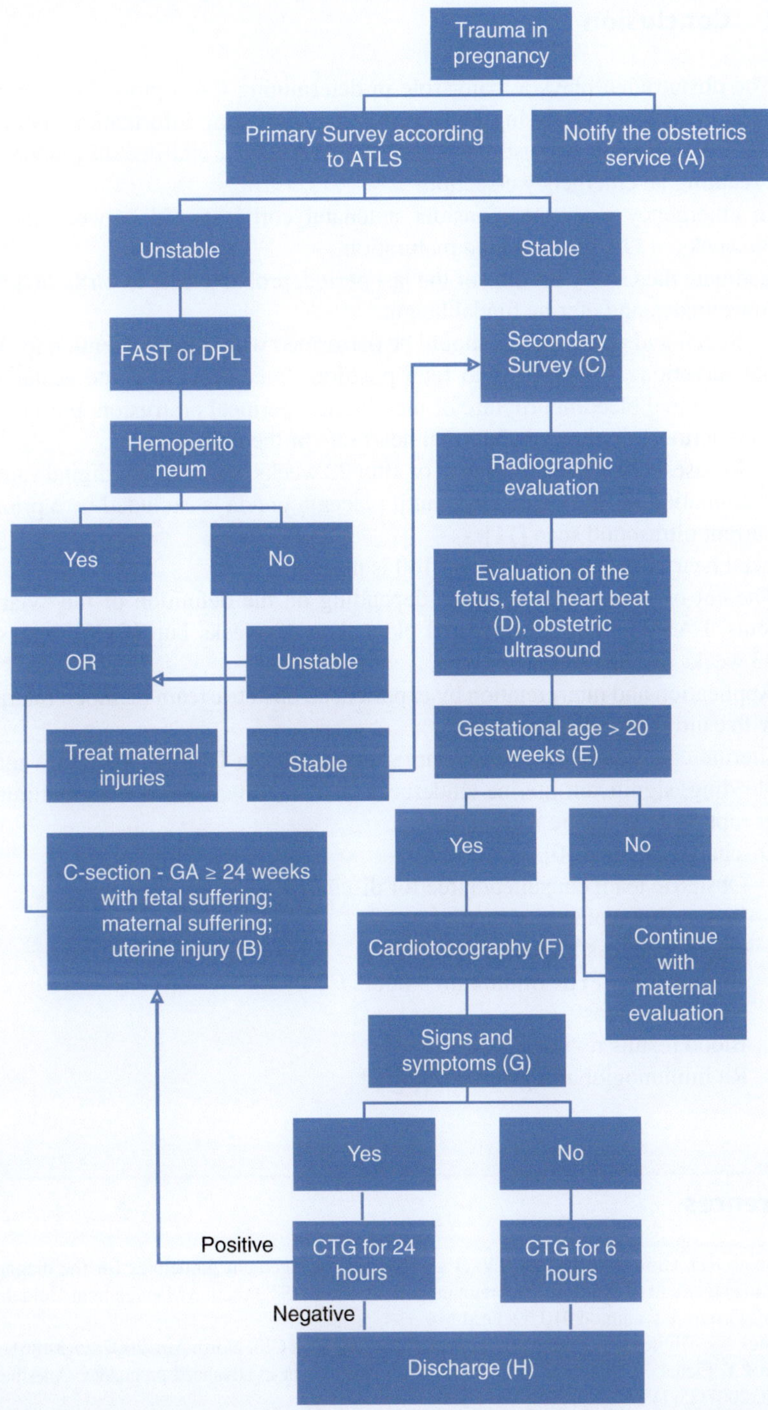

Trauma in pregnancy
Primary Survey according to ATLS
Notify the obstetrics service (A)
Unstable
Stable
FAST or DPL
Secondary Survey (C)
Hemoperitoneum
Radiographic evaluation
Yes
No
Evaluation of the fetus, fetal heart beat (D), obstetric ultrasound
OR
Unstable
Gestational age > 20 weeks (E)
Treat maternal injuries
Stable
Yes
No
C-section - GA ≥ 24 weeks with fetal suffering; maternal suffering; uterine injury (B)
Cardiotocography (F)
Continue with maternal evaluation
Signs and symptoms (G)
Yes
No
Positive
CTG for 24 hours
CTG for 6 hours
Negative
Discharge (H)

39.2 Conclusion

(A) The obstetrician plays a major role in determining GA, optimizing uteroplacental perfusion, assessing fetal well-being, providing information about the risks of radiation exposure and use of medications, and deciding upon and executing an emergency c-section.

(B) In emergency c-section, consider antenatal corticosteroid between 24 and 34 weeks of GA for fetal lung maturation.

(C) Estimate the GA by the date of the last period, probable date of birth, first fetal movements, and uterine fundal height.

Rectal and pelvic exams should be performed with special attention to vaginal secretions, dilatation, and fetal position. Indicatives of acute gestational risk: vaginal bleeding, rupture of membranes, perineal protrusion, presence of contractions, rhythm, or abnormal heart rate of the fetus.

In cases of vaginal bleeding at or after 23 weeks, speculum or digital vaginal examination should be deferred until placenta previa is excluded by a prior or current ultrasound scan [11].

(D) Fetal heartbeat between 110 and 160 is normal.

(E) The cut-off GA for CTG varies depending on the definition of the "viable" fetus. EAST guideline suggested older than 20 weeks but SOGC suggested 23 weeks or older [11].

(F) Application and interpretation by experienced obstetric team member. Interpret with caution at <28 weeks.

(G) Uterine contraction (>1 per 10 min), nonreassuring fetal HR pattern, vaginal bleeding, significant uterine tenderness or irritability, serious maternal injury, or rupture of amniotic membrane.

(H) Discharge criteria [10].
- Obstetric team consulted/agree for discharge
- Reassuring maternal status
- No vaginal loss/bleeding
- Normal CTG/FHR (minimum 4 hours CTG)
- No contractions
- Blood results reviewed
- Rh immunoglobulin given if required

References

1. Barraco RD, Chiu WC, Clancy TV, et al. Practice management guidelines for the diagnosis and management of injury in the pregnant patient: the EAST Practice Management Guidelines Work Group. J Trauma. 2010;69(1):211–4.
2. Cusick SS, Tibbles CD. Trauma in pregnancy. Emerg Med Clin North Am. 2007;25(3):861–72.
3. Meroz Y, Elchalal U, Ginosar Y. Initial trauma management in advanced pregnancy. Anesthesiol Clin. 2007;25(1):117.

4. Einav S, Sela HY, Weiniger CF. Management and outcomes of trauma during pregnancy. Anesthesiol Clin. 2013;31(1):141–56.
5. McAuley DJ. Trauma in pregnancy: anatomical and physiological considerations. Trauma. 2004;6(4):293–300.
6. Epstein FB. Acute abdominal pain in pregnancy. Emerg Med Clin North Am. 1994;12:151–65.
7. Brown S, Mozurkewich E. Trauma during pregnancy. Obstet Gynecol Clin N Am. 2013;40(1):47.
8. Fung Kee Fung K, Eason E, Crane J, et al. Prevention of Rh alloimmunization. J Obstet Gynaecol Can. 2003;25:765–73.
9. Sadro C, Bernstein MP, Kanal KM. Imaging of trauma: part 2, abdominal trauma and pregnancy-a radiologist's guide to doing what is best for the mother and baby. Am J Roentgenol. 2012;199(6):1207–19.
10. Queensland Clinical Guidelines. Trauma in pregnancy. Guideline No. MN14.31-V1-R19. Queensland Health. 2014. Available from: https://www.health.qld.gov.au/__data/assets/pdf_file/0013/140611/g-trauma.pdf.
11. Jain V, Chari R, Maslovitz S, et al. Guidelines for the management of a pregnant trauma patient. J Obstet Gynaecol Can. 2015 Jun;37(6):553–74.

Child Violence

40

Haiana Lopes Cavalheiro, Ana Luisa Bettega,
Carlos F. Oldenburg Neto, Thais Bussyguin,
Maymoona Attiyat, Janaina de Oliveira Poy,
and Antonio Marttos

40.1 Introduction

Abuse or mistreatment is defined by the existence of a subject in superior conditions (age, strength, social or economic position, intelligence, and authority) who commits physical, psychological, or sexual damage, against the will of the victim or by consent obtained by induction or misleading seduction.

Worldwide, almost 3500 children and teenagers die every year by mistreatment. For each death by mistreatment in younger than 15 years, it is estimated that there are 150 cases of physical abuse. The coefficient of mortality by mistreatment is estimated to be 2.2/100,000 for female children and 1.8/100,000 for male children.

H. L. Cavalheiro · A. L. Bettega (✉)
Iwan Collaço Trauma Research Group, Department of Surgery, Hospital do Trabalhador
Trauma Center, Federal University of Parana, Curitiba, Brazil

C. F. Oldenburg Neto · T. Bussyguin
Department of Pediatrics, Hospital do Trabalhador Trauma Center,
Federal University of Parana, Curitiba, Brazil

M. Attiyat
Ryder Trauma Center – Jackson Health System, Miller School of Medicine, University of Miami, Miami, FL, USA

J. de Oliveira Poy
Faculdade de Ciências Médicas de Santos, Santos, São Paulo, Brazil

A. Marttos
William Lehman Injury Research Center, Division of Trauma & Surgical Critical Care,
Dewitt Daughtry Department of Surgery, Leonard M. Miller School of Medicine Miami,
University of Miami, Miami, FL, USA

© Springer Nature Switzerland AG 2020
A. Nasr et al. (eds.), *The Trauma Golden Hour*,
https://doi.org/10.1007/978-3-030-26443-7_40

Although the notification of suspected mistreatment against children and teenagers is legally obligatory, it is estimated that between 10 and 20 cases are not registered to each performed notification. In Curitiba, 1536 cases were notified in 2003 and 3398 in 2006, showing an increase of 54.8%.

Violence against children is classically divided as follows:

- Abuse or physical aggression which consists of the use of physical strength, intentionally or accidentally, by the aggressor aiming to hurt, damage, or even kill the child, leaving or not visible marks.
- Munchausen syndrome by proxy: situation in which the child is brought to medical care due to invented symptoms and/or signs caused by their aggressor.
- Sexual abuse: act of sexual game in which the aggressor is found in a more developed psychosexual state than the child or the teenager.
- Psychological mistreating: every form of rejection, depreciation, discrimination, disrespect, or exaggerated punishment, using the child or teenager to attend the adult's psychic needs.
- Negligence or abandonment: act of omission of the person responsible for the child or teenager in providing the basic needs for their development.

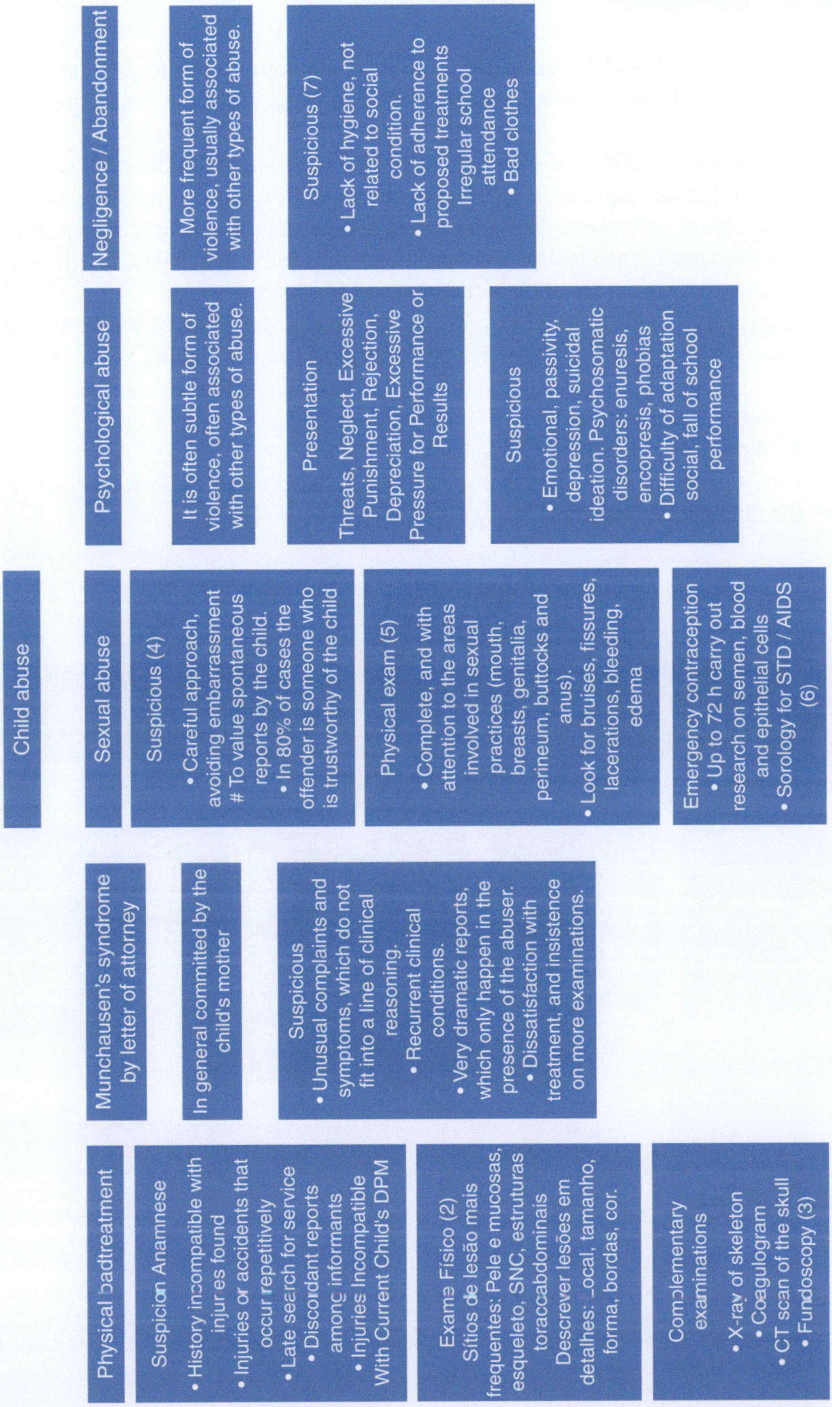

Child abuse

Physical badtreatment

Suspicion Anamnese

- History incompatible with injuries found
- Injuries or accidents that occur repetitively
- Late search for service
- Discordant reports among informants
- Injuries Incompatible With Current Child's DPM

Exame Físico (2)
Sítios de lesão mais frequentes: Pele e mucosas, esqueleto, SNC, estruturas toraccabdominais
Descrever lesões em detalhes: Local, tamanho, forma, bordas, cor.

Complementary examinations

- X-ray of skeleton
- Coagulogram
- CT scan of the skull
- Fundoscopy (3)

Munchausen's syndrome by letter of attorney

In general committed by the child's mother

Suspicious
- Unusual complaints and symptoms, which do not fit into a line of clinical reasoning.
- Recurrent clinical conditions.
- Very dramatic reports, which only happen in the presence of the abuser.
- Dissatisfaction with treatment, and insistence on more examinations.

Sexual abuse

Suspicious (4)

- Careful approach, avoiding embarrassment # To value spontaneous reports by the child.
- In 80% of cases the offender is someone who is trustworthy of the child

Physical exam (5)

- Complete, and with attention to the areas involved in sexual practices (mouth, breasts, genitalia, perineum, buttocks and anus).
- Look for bruises, fissures, lacerations, bleeding, edema

Emergency contraception
- Up to 72 h carry out research on semen, blood and epithelial cells
- Sorology for STD / AIDS (6)

Psychological abuse

It is often subtle form of violence, often associated with other types of abuse.

Presentation
Threats, Neglect, Excessive Punishment, Rejection, Depreciation, Excessive Pressure for Performance or Results

Suspicious

- Emotional, passivity, depression, suicidal ideation. Psychosomatic disorders: enuresis, encopresis, phobias
- Difficulty of adaptation social, fall of school performance

Negligence / Abandonment

More frequent form of violence, usually associated with other types of abuse.

Suspicious (7)

- Lack of hygiene, not related to social condition.
- Lack of adherence to proposed treatments Irregular school attendance
- Bad clothes

40.2 Conclusion

(1) Anamnesis should be empathic, avoiding accusations or pre-judgments and aiming to obtain the maximum amount of information about the nature of the lesions.

(2) Ecchymosis in different stages of evolution, bone lesions in different stages of consolidation, impression left by an instrument of aggression, such as belts, forks, bites, and others, are various indications suggestive of intentional lesion.

(3) Fundoscopy is mandatory in suspected shaken baby syndrome, in which the presence of retinal bleeding is fundamental for the diagnosis.

(4) Approach by an experienced professional avoids repetition of the same questions which can lead to excessive embarrassment of the victims.

(5) There is no need of an expert examination at the legal medical institute for the report of sexual abuse.

(6) HIV prophylaxis with AZT can be indicated.

(7) Low socioeconomic condition should not be used as an attenuating factor for the negligence situation.

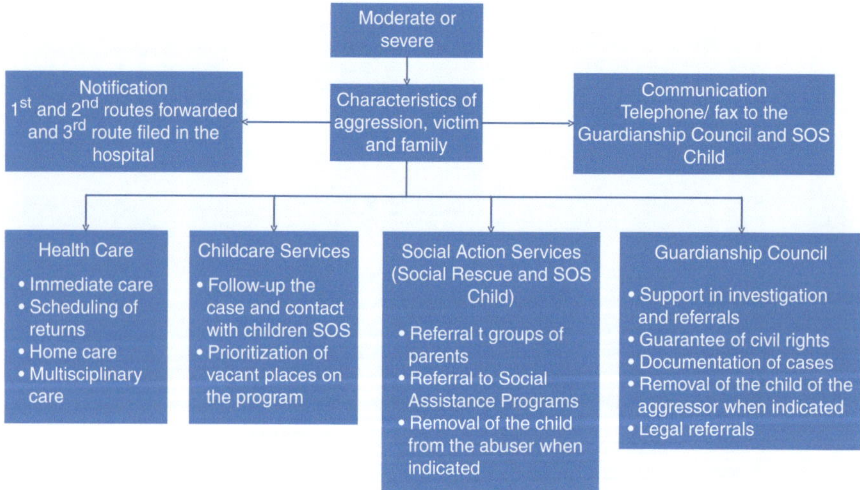

Bibliography

1. Sociedade Brasileira de Pediatria. Guia de Atuação Frente aos Maus-tratos na Infância e na Adolescência. Rio de Janeiro, 2ª edição, 2001.

2. King JW, Mackay M, Sirnick A, with the Canadian Shaken Baby Study Group. Shaken baby syndrome in Canada: clinical characteristics and outcomes of hospital cases. Can Med Assoc J. 2003;168(2):155–8.

3. Camargo DA, Muraro HMS, Costa JCR. Maus-tratos contra crianças e adolescentes em Curitiba, 2003–2006. Prefeitura Municipal de Curitiba, Secretaria Municipal de Saúde, Centro de Epidiemiologia; 2008. p. 1–38.
4. Muraro HMS e colaboradores. Protocolo da Rede de Proteção à Criança e ao Adolescente em Situação de Risco para a Violencia Prefeitura Municipal de Curitiba; 2008. p. 160.
5. Godoy Martins CB. Maus tratos contra crianças e adolescentes. Rev Bras Enfermagem, Brasilia. 2010;63(4):660–5.
6. Ricci LR, Botash, AS, McKenney DM. Child abuse in emergency medicine http://emedicine. medscape.com/article/800657-overview. Accessed on 10/05/12.

Nutritional Therapy in Trauma

41

Alessandra Borges, Rodrigo Furtado Andrade,
Emanuel Antonio Grasselli, Janaina de Oliveira Poy,
Jonathan Parks, D. Dante Yeh, and Patricia Byers

The metabolic response to trauma results in a series of changes culminating in an increase in catabolism, nitrogen depletion, and alterations in glucose and lipid metabolism.

During the *Ebb* phase, immediately following injury, the metabolic rate is maintained at baseline or even decreased. This phase lasts for 1 to 3 days and is followed by the *Flow* phase, which is characterized by an increase in metabolism that is commonly accompanied by catabolism. Nitrogen loss intensifies and, consequently, lean body mass is quickly lost. A previously young and healthy patient suddenly affected by a severe trauma has little time to adapt, and the natural consequence of that is acute disease-related malnutrition.

The primary aim of nutritional therapy in trauma is to minimize this catabolism, avoid malnutrition, or, if the patient is already malnourished, to mitigate its effect on the healing process.

A. Borges · R. F. Andrade
Department of Surgery, Hospital do Trabalhador Trauma Center,
Federal University of Parana, Curitiba, Brazil

E. A. Grasselli
Iwan Collaço Trauma Research Group, Department of Surgery, Hospital do Trabalhador
Trauma Center, Federal University of Parana, Curitiba, Brazil

J. de Oliveira Poy
Faculdade de Ciências Médicas de Santos, Santos, São Paulo, Brazil

J. Parks
Ryder Trauma Center – Jackson Health System, Miami, FL, USA

Miller School of Medicine, University of Miami, Miami, FL, USA

D. D. Yeh (✉) · P. Byers
Division of Trauma Surgery & Critical Care, DeWitt Daughtry Family Department of
Surgery, Miller School of Medicine, University of Miami, Miami, FL, USA
e-mail: dxy154@med.miami.edu

© Springer Nature Switzerland AG 2020
A. Nasr et al. (eds.), *The Trauma Golden Hour*,
https://doi.org/10.1007/978-3-030-26443-7_41

Once the patient has survived the immediate trauma and resuscitation is complete, the need for nutritional support should be determined immediately. The nutritional evaluation of the trauma patient is no different from that of any other surgical patient, and begins with a complete nutritional history, assessing the patient's diet and history of weight loss or weight gain. Patients at low nutritional risk, as determined by the modified NUTRIC score, may be delayed in initiating nutritional support for up to 1 week. Those at high risk should have nutritional support initiated immediately following stabilization.

Next, the patient's nutritional needs should be assessed. If available, indirect calorimetry (IC) should be used to measure resting energy expenditure (REE). If IC is not available, basal energy expenditure (BEE) is determined using several techniques. A simple estimate to start with is 25 kcal/kg/day. The Harris-Benedict equation provides another method of estimation based on the patient's sex, height, weight, and age.

Harris-Benedict equation to estimate basal energy expenditure

$$BEE\,(Male) = 66.5 + \left(13.75 \times weight\ (kg)\right) + \left(5.003 \times height\,(cm)\right) \\ - \left(6.755 \times age\ (years)\right)$$

$$BEE\,(Female) = 655.1 + \left(9.563 \times weight\ (kg)\right) + \left(1.850 \times height\,(cm)\right) \\ - \left(4.676 \times age\ (years)\right)$$

Once BEE is established, a stress factor is added to provide additional nutrition during the period of increased metabolic rate and needs. The stress factor is based on estimates and increased with severity of illness. A typical stress factor for trauma patients ranges from 1.3 to 1.5. For burn patients, it is as high as 2.0.

After determination of the total caloric need, the patient's protein needs are determined. The usual daily protein requirement for a trauma patient is 1.8–2.0 g/kg/day. For patients on continuous renal replacement therapy, the requirement is 2.3–2.5 g/kg/day due to loss of protein across the dialysis membrane.

After determination of the nutritional needs, the route of nutrition is decided. The enteral route is preferred over the parenteral route, as this maintains gut mucosal integrity and avoids the need to establish central venous access required for parenteral nutrition.

Nutritional needs in trauma patients

Clinical status	Estimated nutritional needs, kcal/kg/day	Estimated protein needs, g/kg/day
Moderate trauma	25	1.2–1.5
Severe trauma	20–25	1.5–2.0
Severe TBI (Glasgow <8)		
No paralysis	30	1.2–2,0
With paralysis	25	
Spinal cord trauma with paraplegia	20–22	1.2–1,5
Major burn	25	2.0

Enteral feeding can be delivered via a nasogastric feeding tube to the stomach or more distally to the jejunum. Various tube feed formulas exist with variations in electrolyte, protein, water, and fiber content. Patient comorbidities and fluid goals typically direct the choice of formula. For patients needing enteral feeding access for longer than a few months (e.g., patients with severe traumatic brain injury (TBI)), surgical access can be provided with a gastrostomy or jejunostomy.

For patients who cannot tolerate enteral nutrition due to traumatic injury to the gut, obstruction, ileus, etc., parenteral nutrition (PN) can be provided. Nutrient admixtures should be customized daily. PN can be provided via a central venous catheter or peripherally inserted central catheter (PICC). Administration of these formulas has improved over the last decade, with fewer complications than previously reported. Patients on PN, however, are still susceptible to liver dysfunction, line infection, and hyperglycemia.

Special consideration for providing nutrition to trauma patients also involves the administration of glutamine, arginine, and omega-3 fatty acids. Current recommendations of the American Society of Parenteral and Enteral Nutrition (ASPEN) favors *against* the IV supplementation of glutamine. ASPEN also discourages the use of arginine and fish oil in trauma, TBI, and burn patients. Arginine is contraindicated in sepsis, as it has been associated with increased mortality.

Flowchart 41.1 Nutritional overall plan in polytraumatized patients

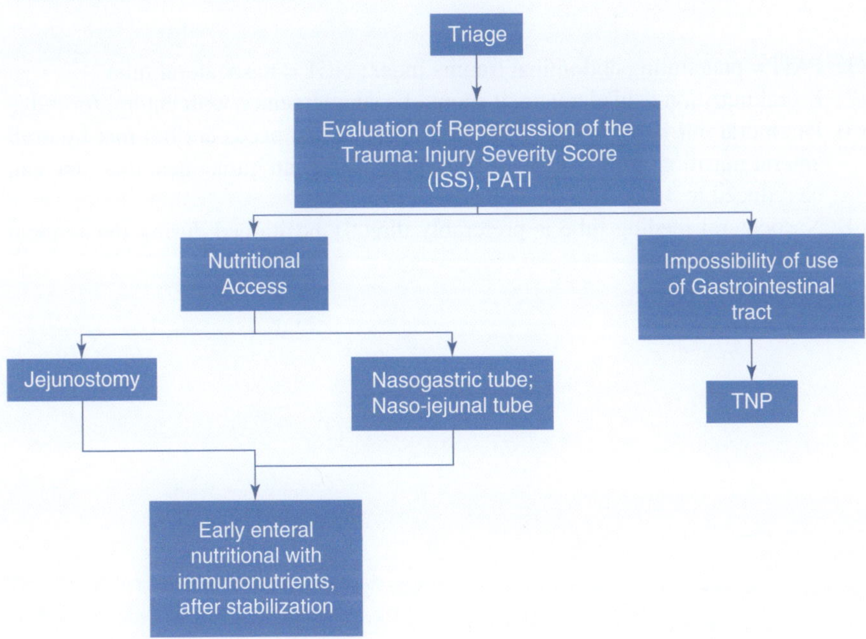

(1) ENT = enteral nutritional therapy; PN = parenteral nutrition
(2) When oral nutrition is allowed, it must be supplemented with adequate enteral formulas.

Flowchart 41.2 Recommendations for penetrating trauma victims

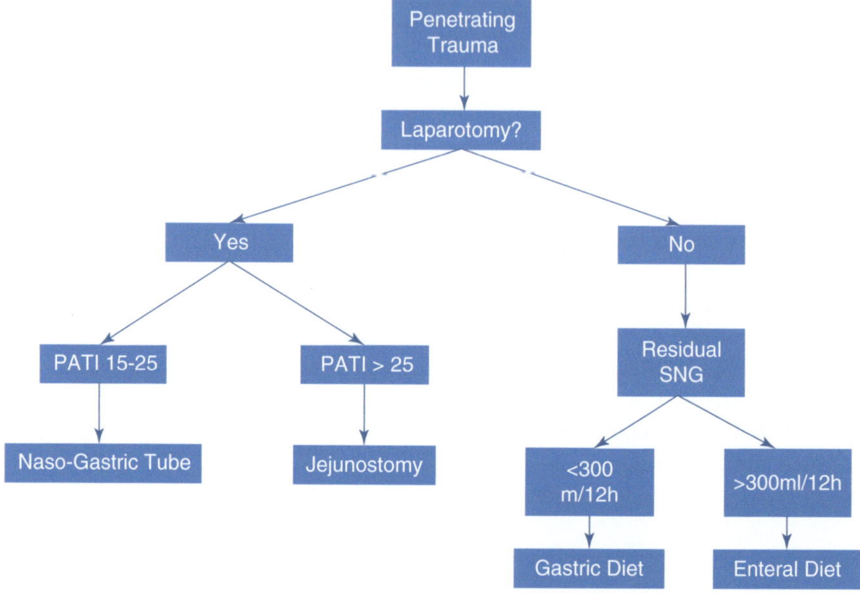

(1) PATI = penetrating abdominal trauma index; NET = nasoenteral tube
(2) If oral nutrition is inadequate, it should be supplemented with enteral formula.
(3) Parenteral nutrition: always indicated if nutritional needs are not met by oral/enteral nutrition after 7 days (according to European guidelines, this time can be reduced to 3 days).
(4) Nasoenteral feeding tube is preferably directly positioned during the surgical intervention.

Flowchart 41.3 Recommendations for blunt trauma victims

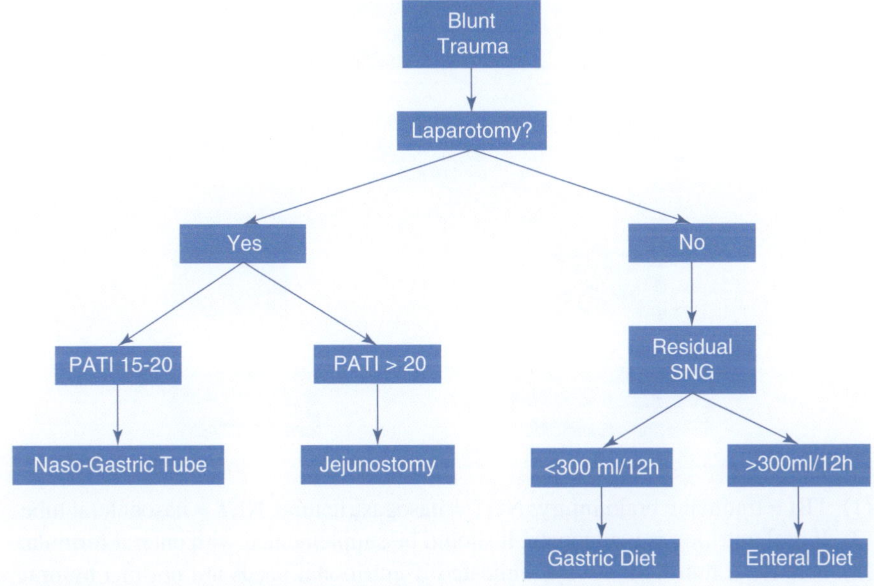

(1) ISS = injury severity score; NET = nasoenteral tube
(2) If oral nutrition is inadequate, it should be supplemented with enteral formula.
(3) Parenteral nutrition: always indicated if nutritional needs are not met by oral/enteral nutrition after 7 days (according to European guidelines, this time can be reduced to 3 days).

Flowchart 41.4 Recommendation for victims of traumatic brain injury

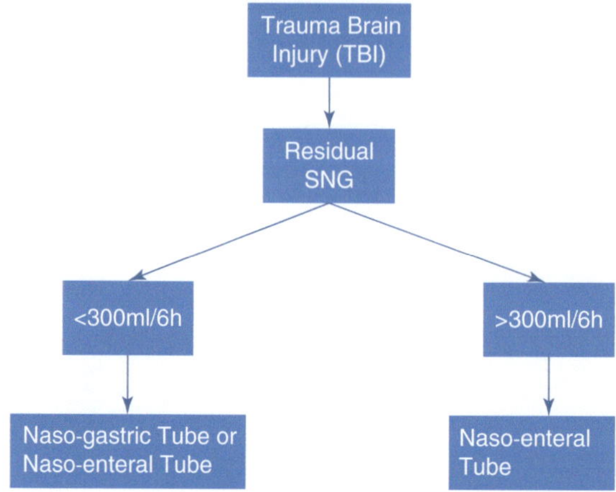

(1) TBI = traumatic brain injury; NGT = nasogastric tube, NET = nasoenteral tube.
(2) If oral nutrition is inadequate, it should be supplemented with enteral formula.
(3) Parenteral nutrition: always indicated if nutritional needs are not met by oral/enteral nutrition after 7 days (according to European guidelines, this time can be reduced to 3 days).

Bibliography

1. ASPEN Board of Directors and the Clinical Guidelines Task Force. Guidelines for the use of parenteral and enteral nutrition in adult and pediatric patients. JPEN J Parenter Enteral Nutr. 2002;26(1 Suppl):1SA–138SA.
2. Braga M, Ljungqvist O, Soeters P, Fearon K, Weimann A, Bozzetti F. ESPEN guidelines on parenteral nutrition: surgery. Clin Nutr. 2009;28(4):378–86.
3. McClave SA, Martindale RG, Vanek VW, et al. Guidelines for the provision and assessment of nutrition support therapy in the adult critically ill patient: Society of Critical Care Medicine (SCCM) and American Society for Parenteral and Enteral Nutrition (A.S.P.E.N.). JPEN J Parenter Enteral Nutr. 2009;33:277–316.
4. Nascimento JEA, Campos ACL, Borges A, Correia MITD, Tavares GM. Terapia Nutricional no Trauma. Em: Projeto Diretrizes, volume IX. São Paulo. Associação Médica Brasileira/Conselho Federal de Medicina; 2011. p. 375–91.
5. Weimann A, Braga M, Harsanyi L, Laviano A, Ljungqvist O, et al. ESPEN guidelines enteral nutrition: surgery including organ transplantation. Clin Nutr. 2006;25:224–44.

Imaging in Trauma

42

Thiago Américo Murakami, Lúcio Eduardo Kluppel, Beatriz Ortis Yazbek, and Antonio Marttos

42.1 Introduction

Along this book, the theme imaging in trauma, mainly in what concerns ultrasound and computed tomography, was extensively cited in the services protocols. This chapter aims to explain in a simple and objective way the main advantages and disadvantages of each one of these methods and the technical approach of ultrasound in the face of an emergency.

Since it emerged as a diagnostic method during the Second World War, ultrasonography was instituted as an important method in the assistance of trauma victims. Initially, it was only used for abdominal exams. However, as long as experience with the method was earned, it came to be used also for thoracic evaluation. In 1997, it received the denomination FAST (Focused Assessment with Sonography for Trauma), and used worldwide until the present time.

T. A. Murakami (✉)
Iwan Collaço Trauma Research Group, Department of Surgery, Hospital do Trabalhador Trauma Center, Federal University of Parana, Curitiba, Brazil

L. E. Kluppel
Department of Radiology, Hospital do Trabalhador Trauma Center, Federal University of Parana, Curitiba, Brazil

B. O. Yazbek
Faculdade de Ciências Médicas de Santos, Santos, São Paulo, Brazil

A. Marttos
William Lehman Injury Research Center, Division of Trauma & Surgical Critical Care, Dewitt Daughtry Department of Surgery, Leonard M. Miller School of Medicine Miami, University of Miami, Miami, FL, USA

© Springer Nature Switzerland AG 2020
A. Nasr et al. (eds.), *The Trauma Golden Hour*,
https://doi.org/10.1007/978-3-030-26443-7_42

Blunt abdominal trauma: FAST × computed tomography

	FAST	Tomography
Stability	Unstable	Stable
Aim	Search free fluid	Search organic injuries
Advantages	Early diagnosis FAST can be repeated Accuracy of 86–97%	Specific to define injury Sensibility of 92–98%
Disadvantages	Operator-dependent Image distortion due to meteorism and subcutaneous emphysema Did not diagnose injuries to the pancreas, intestine, and diaphragm	High cost and duration Use of contrast – Risk of anaphylaxis Did not diagnose injuries to the pancreas, intestine, and diaphragm

42.2 Technique

Transductor: convex – 2.5–3.5 MHz
   Tracking sites:

- Perihepatic space: right posterior axillary line – between 11 and 12 ribs.
- Perisplenic space: left posterior axillary line – between 10 and 11 ribs.
- Pericardium: Transductor on the right side of the xiphoid appendix and left inferior costal ridge.
- Pelvis: Transductor at the midline, above the pubic symphysis.

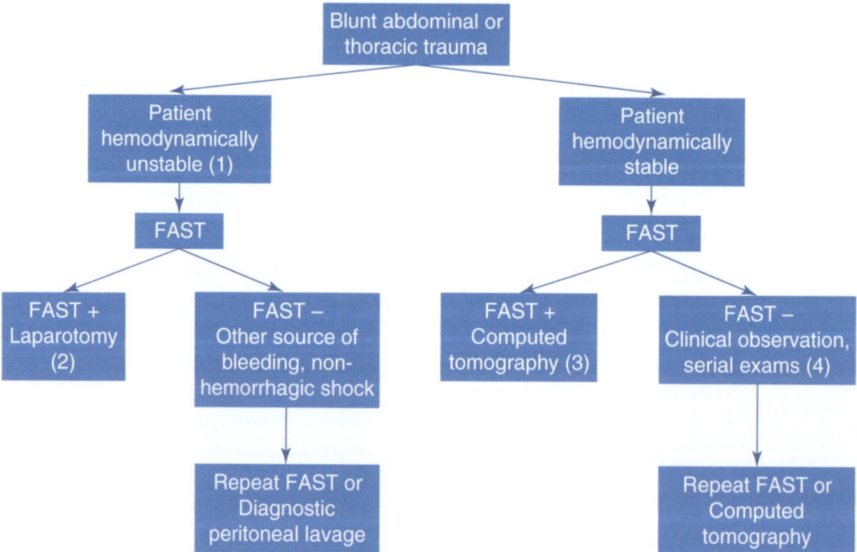

42.3 Conclusion

(1) Blunt abdominal trauma victim who is hemodynamically unstable should be quickly approached by a cheap and sensible method of triage which does not interfere with other procedures. This is the great advantage of FAST. It will document only the presence or absence of free fluid in pericardium, perihepatic space, perisplenic space, and pelvis.

(2) Hemodynamically unstable patients with a negative FAST make us think about other causes of shock. It is worth to remember that although very accurate, as every ultrasound, FAST is operator-dependent . Furthermore, obese patients, with intestinal weather or subcutaneous emphysema, have the exam impaired. Also, injuries of the diaphragm, intestine, and pancreas are not diagnosed by the exam.

(3) Patients with a positive FAST, but hemodynamically stable, always should undergo a computed tomography with intravenous contrast. This exam has an accuracy of 92–98%, providing us with information about the presence of injuries of specific organs, retroperitoneal injuries, and pelvic injuries. It is worth to remember that tomography cannot detect injuries of the diaphragm, intestine, and pancreas. Therefore, a positive FAST in the absence of hepatic or splenic injuries is very suggestive of injury to the gastrointestinal tract or mesentery. From this point, the conduct will be taken according to the grade of impairment found in CT or the patient's clinical change.

(4) In case of hemodynamic stability and negative FAST, it is important to do clinical observation of the patient, be alert to possible changes of the general condition, fall of the blood pressure, or the hematocrit. If any change happens, FAST can be repeated or a CT can be performed.

Bibliography

1. Tsui CL, Fung HT, Chung KL, et al. Focused abdominal sonography for trauma in the emergency department for blunt abdominal trauma. Int J Emerg Med. 2008;1:183–7.
2. Rodriguez C, Barone J, Wilbanks TO, et al. Isolated free fluid on computed tomographic scan in blunt abdominal trauma: a systematic review of incidence and management. J Trauma. 2002;53:79–85.
3. Stengel D, Bauwens K, Sehouli J, Rademacher G, Mutze S, Ekkernkamp A, Porzsolt F. Emergency ultrasound-based algorithms for diagnosing blunt abdominal trauma. Cochrane Database Syst Rev. 2005, 2005;(2):CD004446.
4. Wilson S, Mackay A. Ultrasound in critical care, continuing education in anaesthesia. Critical Care & Pain Advance. 2012;190–94.
5. Advanced Trauma Life Support – American College of Surgeons, 633 N. St. Clair, Chicago, IL 60611, 2004.

Corrections to: The Trauma Golden Hour

Adonis Nasr, Flavio Saavedra Tomasich, Iwan Collaço,
Phillipe Abreu, Nicholas Namias, and Antonio Marttos

Correction to:
A. Nasr et al. (eds.),
The Trauma Golden Hour,
https://doi.org/10.1007/978-3-030-26443-7

The affiliation of co-editors Nicholas Namias and Antonio Marttos was incorrectly updated in the book front matter and this is corrected as follows:

Ryder Trauma Center
Jackson Memorial Hospital
University of Miami
Miami, FL
USA

The corrected online version of this book can be found at
https://doi.org/10.1007/978-3-030-26443-7

© Springer Nature Switzerland AG 2020
A. Nasr et al. (eds.), *The Trauma Golden Hour,*
https://doi.org/10.1007/978-3-030-26443-7_43

Index

© Springer Nature Switzerland AG 2020
A. Nasr et al. (eds.), *The Trauma Golden Hour*,
https://doi.org/10.1007/978-3-030-26443-7

MIX
Papier aus verantwortungsvollen Quellen
Paper from responsible sources
FSC® C105338

If you have any concerns about our products,
you can contact us on
ProductSafety@springernature.com

In case Publisher is established outside the EU,
the EU authorized representative is:
Springer Nature Customer Service Center GmbH
Europaplatz 3, 69115 Heidelberg, Germany

Printed by Libri Plureos GmbH
in Hamburg, Germany